YELLOW-FEVER VACCINATING CENTRES
FOR INTERNATIONAL TRAVEL
Situation as on 1 January 1985

CENTRES DE VACCINATION
CONTRE LA FIÈVRE JAUNE
POUR LES VOYAGES INTERNATIONAUX
Situation au 1er janvier 1985

UN9
WHO
85Y22

WORLD HEALTH ORGANIZATION
ORGANISATION MONDIALE DE LA SANTÉ
GENÈVE
1985

ISBN 92 4 058011 5

PRINTED IN SWITZERLAND
84/6159— Presses Centrales — 8000

CONTENTS

SOMMAIRE

FOREWORD

The International Health Regulations (Article 66, paragraph 4) provide that an international certificate of vaccination against yellow fever is valid only if the vaccine used has been approved by the World Health Organization and if the vaccinating centre has been designated by the health administration for the territory in which the centre is situated. Each Member State is obliged to send a list of such designated centres to WHO.

This booklet contains the names of designated vaccinating centres, and in a few instances of vaccinators, in accordance with the notifications received by the World Health Organization from health administrations. The list of institutes manufacturing yellow-fever vaccines approved by the World Health Organization is published on page 63.

All international certificates of vaccination or revaccination against yellow fever issued by a centre that has subsequently been deleted from the list of designated vaccinating centres remain valid for ten years.

AVANT-PROPOS

Le Règlement sanitaire international (article 66, paragraphe 4) stipule que le certificat international de vaccination contre la fièvre jaune n'est valable que si le vaccin employé a été approuvé par l'Organisation mondiale de la Santé et si le centre de vaccination a été habilité par l'administration sanitaire du territoire dans lequel le centre est situé. Tous les Etats Membres sont tenus d'adresser à l'OMS la liste des centres qu'ils auront ainsi habilités.

La présente brochure contient les noms des centres de vaccination et, dans certains cas, des vaccinateurs habilités, conformément aux notifications communiquées à l'Organisation mondiale de la Santé par les administrations sanitaires. La liste des instituts préparant un vaccin contre la fièvre jaune approuvé par l'Organisation mondiale de la Santé figure à la page 63.

Tous les certificats internationaux de vaccination ou de revaccination contre la fièvre jaune qui ont été délivrés par un centre supprimé par la suite de la liste des centres de vaccination habilités restent valables pendant dix ans.

LIST OF DESIGNATED VACCINATING CENTRES

LISTE DES CENTRES DE VACCINATION HABILITÉS

ALGERIA
ALGÉRIE

Alger—
- Institut Pasteur d'Algérie, rue du Docteur Laveran, El-Annasser
- Contrôle sanitaire aux Frontières, Santé maritime, quai Nord, Port d'Alger

ANGOLA

Delegado de Saúde

Bailundo
Benguela
Caála
Cabinda
Camacupa
Capelongo
Cela
Dondo
Gabela
Ganda
Ganguelas
Lobito
Luanda
Malange
Maquela do Zombo
Menongue
Moçâmedes
Nóqui
Nova Lisboa
Novo Redondo
Porto Alexandre
Porto Amboim
Quibala

Sá da Bandeira
S. António do Zaire
S. Salvador do Congo
Suarimo
Silva Porto
Uíge
Vila Luso
Vila Pereira d'Eça
Vila Salazar
Vila Teixeira de Sousa

ARGENTINA
ARGENTINE

Unidades Sanitarias dependientes de la Dirección Nacional de Sanidad de Fronteras y Transportes del Ministerio de Salud Pública y Medio Ambiente

Bahía Blanca (A)
Bernarco de Irigoyen (A)
Buenos Aires (A)
Buenos Aires — Aeroparque (A)
Clorinda (B)
Comodoro Rivadavia (B)
Concepción del Uruguay (B)
Córdoba (A)
Corrientes (A)
Ezeiza (A)
Formosa (A)
Gualeguaychú (B)
Iguazú (B)
Ituzaingó (A)
Jujuy (B)
La Plata (B)
La Quiaca (A)
Mar del Plata (B)
Mendoza (A)
Neuquén (A)

Note
The symbol • is used before the name of a centre simply to help readers locate the required centre when there is more than one in a particular town. Otherwise it does not have any special signifiance.

L'emploi du symbole • devant le nom d'un centre a simplement pour but d'aider le lecteur à repérer le centre requis lorsqu'il existe plusieurs centres dans une même ville. Ce symbole n'a par ailleurs aucune signification spéciale.

ARGENTINA *(continued)*
ARGENTINE *(suite)*

Paso de los Libres (B)
Posadas (A)
Puerto Deseado (B)
Puerto Madryn (B)
Puyehué (B)
Quequén (B)
Resistencia (A)
Río Gallegos (A)
Río Mayo (B)
Río Turbio (A)
Rosario (A)
Salta (B)
Salto Grande (A)
Salvador Mazza (A)
San Antonio Este (B)
San Carlos de Bariloche (B)
San Juan (B)
San Nicolás (B)
Santa Fé (B)
Tucumán (A)
Ushuaía (A)

AUSTRALIA
AUSTRALIE

The Commonwealth Department of Health (through its regional offices in each state and territory)

Le Ministère fédéral de la Santé (par l'intermédiaire de ses services régionaux dans chaque état et territoire)

New South Wales

Richmond —
 No. 3 Royal Australian Air Force Hospital, RAAF Base

AUSTRIA
AUTRICHE

Bregenz —
 Amt der Vorarlberger Landesregierung
 Medizinische Abteilung
Graz —
 Amt der Steiermärkischen Landesregierung

Innsbruck —
 Amt der Tiroler Landesregierung
Klagenfurt —
 Amt der Kärntner Landesregierung
Linz —
 Amt der Oberösterr. Landesregierung
Salzburg —
 Amt der Salzburger Landesregierung
Wien —
 • Amt der Niederösterr. Landesregierung
 • IAEA-UNIDO Joint Medical Service
 • Institut für Spezifische Prophylaxie und Tropenmedizin der Universität
 • Magistrat der Stadt, Mag. Abt. 15
Wiener Neustadt —
 Magistrat Wiener Neustadt, Gesundheitsamt
Zwettl —
 Bezirkshauptmannschaft Zwettl, Gesundheitsabteilung

BAHAMAS

Grand Bahama
Freeport —
 District Medical Officer

New Providence
Nassau —
 Medical Officer of Health

BAHRAIN
BAHREÏN

Bahrain —
 • Directorate of Public Health
 • Health Office, Bahrain International Airport

BANGLADESH

Chalna —
 Port Health Department
Chittagong —
 Port Health Department
Dhaka —
 Airport Health Department

BARBADOS
BARBADE

Bridgetown —
Enmore Health Centre

BELGIUM
BELGIQUE

Antwerpen (Anvers) —
- Gezondheidsdienst der Havens
- Gezondheidsinspectie van Antwerpen
- Institut de Médecine tropicale Prince Léopold — Instituut voor Tropische Geneeskunde Prins Leopold
- Pool der Zeelieden, Antwerpen — Seamen's Pool, Antwerp

Brugge (Bruges) —
Gezondheidsinspectie van West-Vlaanderen

Bruxelles —
- Centre médical du Ministère des Affaires étrangères — Medische Centrum van het Ministerie van Buitenlandse Zaken
- Section de Médecine tropicale de la Direction générale des Service de Santé — Adeling Tropische Geneeskunde van de Algemene directie der Gezondheidsdiensten
- Service médical, Sabena — Medische dienst, Sabena
- Service sanitaire des Ports et Aéroports — Gezondheidsdienst der havens en luchthavens

Charleroi —
Inspection de l'Hygiène du Hainaut

Gent (Gand) —
Gezondheidsinspectie van Oost-Vlaanderen

Hasselt —
Gezondheidsinspectie van Limburg

Jambes —
Inspection de l'Hygiène de Namur

Libramont —
Inspection de l'Hygiène du Luxembourg

Liège —
Inspection de l'Hygiène de Liège

Mons —
Inspection de l'Hygiène du Hainaut

BELIZE

Government Hospital

Belize
Cayo
Corozal
Punta Corda
Stann Creek

BENIN
BÉNIN

Cotonou —
Service d'Hygiène

Porto Novo —
Service d'Hygiène

BERMUDA
BERMUDES

Hamilton —
Public Health Department

BOLIVIA
BOLIVIE

La Paz —
División de Enfermedades Transmisibles, Ministerio de Salud Pública

Santa Cruz de la Sierra —
Servicio de Fiebre Amarilla, División de Enfermedades Transmisibles

BOTSWANA

Francistown—
Jubilee Hospital

Gaborone —
Princess Marina Hospital

BOTSWANA *(continued, suite)*

Ghanzi —
  Ghanzi Health Centre
Mahalapye —
  Mahalapye Hospital
Maun —
  Maun General Hospital
Molepolole —
  Scottish Livingstone Hospital
Lobatse —
  Athlone Hospital
Selebi-Phikwe —
  Selebi-Phikwe Government Hospital
Serowe —
  Sekgoma Memorial Hospital

BRAZIL
BRÉSIL

Rio de Janeiro — Rio de Janeiro —
  Inspetoria de Saúde dos Portos, Praça
  Marechal Âncora
Rio Grande do Sul — Porto Alegre —
  Centre de Saúde No. 2 da Secretaria
  Estadual de Saúde
São Paulo — Campinas —
  Inspetoria Seccional, Aeroporto Inter-
  nacional de Viracopos

*Inspetoria de Saúde dos Portos, Aeroportos
e Fronteiras (Divisão Nacional de Vigilân-
cia Sanitária de Portos, Aeroportos e Fronteiras)*

Acre — Rio Branco
Alagoas — Maceió
Amapá — Macapá
Amazonas — Manaus
Bahia — Salvador
Ceará — Fortaleza
Distrito Federal — Brasília
Espírito Santo — Vitória
Maranhão — São Luiz
Mato Grosso — Cuiabá
Mato Grosso do Sul —
  Campo Grande
  Corumba

Pará — Bélem
Paraíba — João Pessoa
Paraná — Curitiba
Pernambuco — Recife
Rio de Janeiro — Rio de Janeiro
Rio Grande do Norte — Natal
Rondônia — Porto Velho
Roraima — Boa Vista
Santa Catarina — Itajaí
São Paulo — São Paulo
Sergipe — Aracaju

*Superintendência de Campanhas de Saúde
Pública (SUCAM)*

Bahia — Ilhéus
Goiás — Goiânia
Minas Gerais —
  Belo Horizonte
  Uberaba
Piauí — Teresina
Acre — Rio Branco-Boa Vista
Rio de Janeiro — Niterói
Rio Grande do Sul —
  Porto Alegre
  Santa Maria
Santa Catarina — Florianópolis
São Paulo — Santos

Inspetoria Seccional do Pôrto Marítimo

Bahia — Ilhéus
Paraná — Paranaguá
Rio de Janeiro — Angra dos Reis
Rio Grande do Sul — Rio Grande
Santa Catarina — São Francisco do Sul
São Paulo —
  Santos
  São Sebastião

BRUNEI DARUSSALAM
BRUNÉI DARUSSALAM

Bandar Seri Begawan —
  Raja Istero Anak Saleha Hospital
Seria —
  Panaga Hospital, B.S.P. Co. Ltd.

BULGARIA
BULGARIE

Bourgas —
 Station sanitaire et épidémiologique
Sofia —
 Station sanitaire et épidémiologique
Varna —
 Station sanitaire et épidémiologique

BURKINA FASO

Bobo-Dioulasso —
 Ambulance
Ouagadougou —
 • Secteur No. 1 du Service
  des Grandes Endémies, Médecin-
  chef
 • Service d'Hygiène, Médecin-chef

BURMA
BIRMANIE

Rangoon —
 National Health Laboratory, 35 Stewart
 Road

BURUNDI

Bujumbura —
 Service de l'Hygiène publique
Kitega —
 Service médical
Ngozi —
 Service médical

CAMEROON
CAMEROUN

Bafoussam —
 Section provinciale de la Médecine préventive et de l'Hygiène publique de
 l'Ouest

Bamenda —
 Section provinciale de la Médecine pré-
 ventive et de l'Hygiène publique du
 Nord-Ouest
Bertoua —
 Section provinciale de la Médecine pré-
 ventive et de l'Hygiène publique de
 l'Est
Douala —
 Section provinciale de la Médecine pré-
 ventive et de l'Hygiène publique du Lit-
 toral
Ebolowa —
 Section provinciale de la Médecine pré-
 ventive et de l'Hygiène publique du
 Centre
Garoua —
 Section provinciale de la Médecine pré-
 ventive et de l'Hygiène publique du
 Nord
Kousseri —
 Section départementale de la Médecine
 préventive et rurale du Logone et
 Chari
Limbe —
 Section provinciale de la Médecine pré-
 ventive et de l'Hygiène publique du Sud-
 Ouest
Mamfé —
 Section départementale de la Médecine
 préventive et rurale de la Manyu
Maroua —
 Section provinciale de la Médecine pré-
 ventive et de l'Hygiène publique de
 l'Extrême-Nord
Mokolo —
 Section départementale de la Médecine
 préventive et rurale de Mayo/Tsanaga
Ngaoundere —
 Section provinciale de la Médecine pré-
 ventive et de l'Hygiène publique de
 l'Adamaoua
Yaoundé —
 • Centre Pasteur
 • Section provinciale de la Médecine
  préventive et de l'Hygiène publique
  du Centre

CANADA

Alberta

Calgary —
International Travel Immunization
Clinic, Health Sciences Centre
Edmonton —
Central Clinic

British Columbia

Lazo —
Base Surgeon, Canadian Forces Base,
Comox *(military personnel only — personnel militaire seulement)*
Prince George —
Northern Interior Health Unit
Vancouver —
Zone Director, Medical Services, Health
and Welfare Canada
Vedder Crossing —
Base Surgeon, Canadian Forces Base,
Chilliwack *(military personnel only — personnel militaire seulement)*
Vernon —
North Okanagan Health Unit
Victoria —
● Base Surgeon, Canadian Forces Base,
Esquimalt, FMO Victoria
● Zone Director, Medical Services,
Health and Welfare Canada

Manitoba

Winnipeg —
Regional Director, Medical Services,
Health and Welfare Canada

New Brunswick

Saint John —
District Medical Health Officer

Newfoundland

St. John's —
Officer-in-Charge, Medical Services,
Health and Welfare Canada

Nova Scotia

Cornwallis —
Base Surgeon, Canadian Forces Base
(military personnel only — personnel militaire seulement)
Halifax —
● Canadian Forces Hospital
● Medical Officer-in-Charge, Medical
Services, Health and Welfare
Canada
Sydney —
Cape Breton Health Unit, Prince
Street

Ontario

Astra —
Base Surgeon, Canadian Forces Base
Kingston —
Base Clinic, Canadian Forces Base
London —
University Hospital, Immunization
Clinic
Midhurst —
Simcoe County District Health Unit,
County Administration Centre
Ottawa —
Regional Director, Overseas Region,
Medical Services, Health and Welfare
Canada
Sudbury —
Medical Officer of Health, Sudbury and
District Health Unit
Thunder Bay —
Lake Superior Health Centre, Medical
Services, Health and Welfare Canada
Toronto —
● Air Canada Medical Clinic, Toronto
AMF
● Canadian National Railways Medical
Clinic
● Toronto General Hospital, Travel and
Inoculation Clinic
● Zone Director, Medical Services,
Health and Welfare Canada

Prince Edward Island

Charlottetown —
Division of Nursing, Department of
Health and Social Services

Québec
Chicoutimi —
  Dr Paul Desmeules, Département de Santé communautaire, Clinique de vaccination des voyageurs
Dorval —
  Air Canada Medical Services, Air Canada Base
Montréal —
  • Clinique médicale du Chemin de Fer Canadien National
  • Clinique de vaccination des voyageurs, Département de Santé communautaire
Québec —
  Département de Santé communautaire, Hôpital du Saint-Sacrement
Richelieu —
  Hôpital militaire, Base des Forces canadiennes, Saint-Jean *(personnel militaire seulement — military personnel only).*
Rimouski —
  Centre local des Services communautaires de l'Estuaire
Sherbrooke —
  Clinique du Voyageur international, Département de Santé communautaire, Centre hospitalier universitaire

Saskatchewan
Regina —
  Medical Officer of Health, City Health Department
Saskatoon —
  Medical Health Officer, City of Saskatoon
In Europe —
  Canadian Forces, Europe Medical Centre, Lahr, Federal Republic of Germany

CAPE VERDE
CAP-VERT

Praîa — ·
  Delegado de Saúde
Sal —
  Delegado de Saúde
São Vicente —
  Delegado de Saúde

CENTRAL AFRICAN REPUBLIC
RÉPUBLIQUE CENTRAFRICAINE

Bangui —
  • Hôpital
  • Institut Pasteur
Bouar —
  Infirmerie de garnison

CHAD
TCHAD

Abéché —
  Secteur médico-sanitaire Nº 5
Ati —
  Secteur médico-sanitaire Nº 6
Bongor —
  Secteur médico-sanitaire Nº 2
Moundou —
  Secteur médico-sanitaire Nº 3
N'Djamena —
  • Direction du Service des Grandes Endémies
  • Secteur médico-sanitaire Nº 1
Sarh —
  Secteur médico-sanitaire Nº 4

CHANNEL ISLANDS
ILES ANGLO-NORMANDES

Guernsey (Guernesey) —
  St. Peter Port —
  Health Department, Lukis House
Jersey —
  St. Helier —
  • Medical Officer of Health
  • Health Centre, General Hospital, Newgate Street

CHILE
CHILI

Antofagasta —
  Jefatura Zonal
Concepción —
  Centro de Salud Concepción
Magallanes —
  Centro de Salud Punta Arenas

CHILE *(continued)*
CHILI *(suite)*

Santiago —
  Centro de Salud San Borja, Vacunatorio
  Internacional
Valparaiso —
  Centro de Salud Almendral
  Centro de Salud Viña del Mar

CHINA
CHINE

Quarantine Service — Service de Quarantaine

Beihai
Beijing
Chengdu
Chenglingji
Chongqing
Dalian
Dandong
Erlian
Fuzhou
Gongbei
Guangzhou
Guilin
Haikou
Hangzhou
Harbin
Heihe
Hekou
Jian
Jiujiang
Kunming
Lianyungang
Manzhouli
Nanjing
Nanning
Nantong Port
Ningbo
Pingxiang
Qingdao
Qinhuangdao
Shanghai
Shantou
Shenyang
Shenzhen
Suifenhe

Tianjin
Tumen
Wuhu
Wulumuqi
Wenzhou
Xiamen
Xian
Yantai
Yingkou
Zhanjiang
Zhanjiang Port
Zhangmu

COLOMBIA
COLOMBIE

Barranquilla —
  Sanidad Portuaria
Bogotá —
  Aeropuerto Eldorado, Sanidad Portuaria, Instituto Nacional de Salud
Bucaramanga —
  Dirección Departamental de Higiene y Centro de Higiene
Buenaventura —
  Sanidad Portuaria
Cali —
  Dirección Departamental de Higiene
Cartagena —
  Sanidad Portuaria
Cúcuta —
  Dirección Departamental de Higiene y Centro de Higiene
Medellín —
  Secretaría de Higiene

COMOROS
COMORES

Anjouan —
  Hôpital de Nombo
Grande Comore —
  Hôpital de Moroni
Mayotte —
  Hôpital de Dzaoudzi
Mohéli —
  Hôpital de Fomboni

Countries or Areas with Yellow-Fever Vaccinating Centres

66

Pays ou zones dotés de centres de vaccination contre la fièvre jaune

Oulu Province

Ämmänsaari
Haapajärvi
Haapavesi
Haukipudas
Kajaani
Kalajoki
Kempele
Kuhmo
Kuusamo
Liminka
Muhos
Nivala
Oulainen
Oulu
Pudasjärvi
Pulkkila
Puolanka
Pyhäsalmi
Raahe
Ristijärvi
Sotkamo
Taivalkoski
Vaala
Vuolijoki
Ylivieska

Pohjois-Karjala Province

Eno
Hammaslahti
Ilomantsi
Joensuu
Juuka
Kitee
Kontiolahti
Lieksa
Liperi
Outokumpu
Porokylä
Tohmajärvi

Turku and Pori Province

Eura
Hämeenkyrö
Harjavalta
Ikaalinen
Kaarina
Kankaanpää
Kimito

Kokemäki
Laitila
Lauttakylä
Lavia
Lieto
Loimaa
Luvia
Mouhijärvi
Mynämäki
Naantali
Noormarkku
Nousiainen
Paimio
Pargas
Parkano
Perniö
Pori
Raisio
Rauma
Riihikoski
Rusko
Salo
Säkylä
Turku
Uusikaupunki
Vammala
Vanha-Ulvila
Vehmaa

Uusimaa Province

Ekenäs
Espoo
Hanko
Helsinki
Hyrylä
Hyvinkää
Järvenpää
Karis
Karkkila
Kauniainen
Kerava
Kirkkonummi
Lohja
Lovisa
Mäntsälä
Nikkilä
Nurmijärvi
Orimattila
Porvoo
Vantaa
Vihti

FINLAND (continued)
FINLANDE (suite)

Vaasa Province

Ähtäri
Alajärvi
Alavus
Härmä
Ilmajoki
Isokyrö
Jakobstad
Jalasjärvi
Kannus
Kauhajoki
Kauhava
Kokkola
Kristiinankaupunki
Kurikka
Lappajärvi
Lapua
Närpes
Nykarleby
Oravainen
Övermalax
Seinäjoki
Smedsby
Terjärvi
Teuva
Tunkkari
Vaasa

FRANCE

Angers —
 Centre hospitalier régional
Bastia (Corse) —
 Bureau municipal d'Hygiène
Bayonne —
 Centre hospitalier
Besançon —
 Centre hospitalier régional
Bordeaux —
 • Centre de Vaccination de la Direction
   départementale de l'Action sanitaire
   et social
 • Hôpital d'Instruction des Armées
   Robert Picqué

Brest —
 Hôpital des Armées Clermont-Tonnerre
Caen —
 Centre hospitalier et universitaire (Service du Professeur Villey)
Clermont-Ferrand —
 Hôpital Saint-Jacques
Dijon —
 Centre hospitalier régional
Grenoble —
 Centre hospitalier régional
Le Havre —
 Centre hospitalier
Lille —
 Institut Pasteur
Lyon —
 • Bureau municipal d'Hygiène
 • Hôpital d'Instruction des Armées
   Desgenettes
 • Institut Pasteur
Marseille —
 • Bureau municipal d'Hygiène
 • Hôpital d'Instruction des Armées
   Laveran
 • Hôpital Houphouët-Boigny
Montpellier —
 Institut Bouisson Bertrand
Nancy —
 Hôpital des Armées Sédillot
Nantes —
 Centre hospitalier régional
Nice —
 • Aéroport de Nice — Côte d'Azur, Bloc
   médico-social
 • Centre hospitalier régional
Orly —
 Service du Contrôle sanitaire aux Frontières (Aéroport Orly Sud)
Paris —
 • Centre Edison, 44 rue Charles
   Moureu
 • Centre médico-social de l'Association
   paritaire d'Action sociale du Bâtiment
   et des Travaux publics de la Région
   parisienne (APAS), 52 avenue Michel
   Bizot
 • Hôpital Claude Bernard, 10 av. de la
   Porte-d'Aubervilliers
 • Hôpital de la Salpêtrière (Service du
   Professeur Gentillini)

- Institut Pasteur
- Service médical, Compagnie Air France
- Service médical, UNESCO

Poitiers —
Centre hospitalier régional
Puteaux —
Union de Transports aériens, 50 rue Arago
Reims —
Centre hospitalier régional (Service des Maladies infectieuses)
Rennes —
Hôpital des Armées Ambroise-Paré
Roissy-en-France —
Service du Contrôle sanitaire aux Frontières (Aéroport Charles de Gaulle)
Rouen —
Centre hospitalier régional, Laboratoire central
Saint-Mandé —
Hôpital d'Instruction des Armées Bégin
Strasbourg —
Institut d'Hygiène, Centre hospitalier
Toulon —
Hôpital d'Instruction des Armées Sainte-Anne
Toulouse —
Centre hospitalier régional de Purpan
Tours —
Centre hospitalier régional
Troyes —
Centre hospitalier général

Guadeloupe

Pointe-à-Pitre —
Institut Pasteur

Guyane française (French Guiana)

Cayenne —
Institut Pasteur

Réunion (Reunion)

Saint-Denis —
Laboratoire du Centre hospitalier de Belle-Pierre Saint-Denis

FRENCH POLYNESIA
POLYNÉSIE FRANÇAISE

Ile de Tahiti
Papeete —
Centre de vaccination contre la fièvre jaune, Service d'Hygiène et de Salubrité publique du Territoire

FRENCH SOUTHERN AND ANTARCTIC TERRITORIES
TERRES AUSTRALES ET ANTARCTIQUES FRANÇAISES

Centre médical

Kerguelen —
Nouvelle Amsterdam
Terre Adélie

GABON

Franceville —
Secteur N° 2 du Service des Grandes Endémies
Koulamoutou —
Secteur N° 7 du Service des Grandes Endémies
Lambaréné —
Secteur N° 3 du Service des Grandes Endémies
Libreville —
- Secteur N° 1 du Service des Grandes Endémies
- Service Urbain d'Hygiène
Makokou —
Secteur N° 6 du Service des Grandes Endémies
Mouila —
Secteur N° 4 du Service des Grandes Endémies
Oyem —
Secteur N° 9 du Service des Grandes Endémies
Port-Gentil —
Secteur N° 8 du Service des Grandes Endémies
Tchibanga —
Secteur N° 5 du Service des Grandes Endémies

GAMBIA
GAMBIE

Banjul —
  Health Office
Bansang —
  Provincial Hospital
Fajara —
  Medical Research Council Laboratories

GERMAN DEMOCRATIC REPUBLIC
RÉPUBLIQUE DÉMOCRATIQUE ALLEMANDE

Berlin —
● Betriebspoliklinik im Haus der Ministerien
● Medizinischer Dienst des Verkehrswesens der DDR, Direktion Zivile Luftfahrt, Flughafen Berlin-Schönefeld, Impfstelle
● Städtisches Klinikum Berlin-Buch, Zentrale Impfstelle des Magistrats von Berlin, Hauptstadt der DDR, tropenmedizinischpoliklinische Abteilung
Cottbus —
  Bezirkskrankenhaus, Innere Poliklinik, Untersuchungs- und Impfstelle für Auslandsreisende
Dresden —
  Bezirkskrankenhaus Dresden-Friedrichstadt, Untersuchungs- und Impfstelle für Auslandsreisende
Erfurt —
  Rat der Stadt Erfurt, Zentrales Impfwesen, Fischmarkt 19/20
Frankfurt/Oder —
  Bezirkskrankenhaus Frankfurt/Oder, Medizinische Poliklinik Untersuchungs- und Impfstelle für Auslandsreisende
Karl-Marx-Stadt —
  Bezirkskrankenhaus Karl-Marx-Stadt, Klinik für Infektionskrankheiten
Leipzig —
  Bezirkskrankenhaus St. Georg, Untersuchungs- und Impfstelle für Auslandsreisende

Hafenarzt

Rostock
Sassnitz
Stralsund
Wismar

GERMANY, FEDERAL REPUBLIC OF
ALLEMAGNE, RÉPUBLIQUE FÉDÉRALE D'

Aachen —
  Abteilung Med. Mikrobiologie der Technischen Hochschule (Zulassung Nr. 10)
Augsburg —
  Städtisches Gesundheitsamt (Bavaria Vaccinating Centre No. 5)
Aurich —
  Staatliches Medizinaluntersuchungsamt (Niedersachsen Vaccinating Centre No. OL 3)
Baden-Baden —
  DRK-Blutspendedienst (Baden-Württemberg Vaccinating Centre No. 4)
Bochum —
● Hygiene-Institut der Ruhr-Universität (Zulassung Nr. 16)
● Dr Feodora Hoffmann, Marienplatz 2 (Zulassung Nr. 20)
Bonn —
● Auswärtiges Amt — Impfstation (Zulassung Nr. 2)
● Hygiene-Institut der Universität (Zulassung Nr. 1)
Brake —
  Staatliches Gesundheitsamt Wesermarsch
Braunschweig —
  Staatliches Medizinaluntersuchungsamt (Niedersachsen Vaccinating Centre No. Br. 1)
Bremen —
  Hafengesundheitsamt
Bremerhaven —
  Hafengesundheits- und Quarantäneamt
Dortmund —
  Dr H. Reinicke, Hovelstr. 8 (Zulassung Nr. 3)

Duisburg —
Dr E. Oppermann, Landfermann-
strasse 1 (Zulassung Nr. 12)
Düsseldorf —
- Gesundheitsamt — Hafen- und Flug-
hafenärztlicher Dienst (Zulassung Nr.
18)
- Institut für Hygiene der Universität
(Zulassung Nr. 4)
Emden —
Hafenarzt
Erlangen —
- Institut für Umwelthygiene und Prä-
ventivmedizin der Universität (Bava-
ria Vaccinating Centre No. 16)
- Kinder- und Poliklinik der Universi-
tät (Bavaria Vaccinating Centre
No. 15)
Essen —
Institut für Med. Virologie und Immu-
nologie des Universitätsklinikums (Zu-
lassung Nr. 6)
Frankfurt/Main —
- Hygiene-Institut der Universität
- Stadtgesundheitsamt — Flughafen-
arzt
Freiburg —
Staatliches Gesundheitsamt (Baden-
Württemberg Vaccinating Centre
No. 6)
Gelsenkirchen —
Dr O. Schmidt, Pawickerstrasse 30
(Zulassung Nr. 14)
Giessen —
Hygiene-Institut der Universität, Zen-
trum für Ökologie
Göttingen —
Hygiene-Institut der Universität, Viro-
logische Abteilung (Niedersachsen Vac-
cinating Centre No. Hi 1)
Gütersloh —
Dr K.H. Bründel, Carl Bertelsmann-
Strasse 161 (Zulassung Nr. 21)
Hagen —
Dr Walburga Spannaus, Grabenstrasse
35 (Zulassung Nr. 7)
Hamburg —
- Bernard-Nocht-Institut für Schiffs-
und Tropenkrankheiten, Bernard-
Nocht-Strasse 74
- Hafenärztlicher Dienst, Baumwall 7

- Institut für Impfwesen und Virologie,
Hinrichsenstrasse 1
- Institut für Med. Mikrobiologie und
Immunologie am Universitäts-Kran-
kenhaus Eppendorf, Martinistrasse
52
- Medizinische Untersuchungsstelle I
der Bundeswehr (Hamburg Vaccina-
ting Centre No. 1)
- Dr A. Melenkeit, Johannisbollwerk 6
(Hamburg Vaccinating Centre
No. 4)
- Dr K. Sievers, Schaartor 1(Hamburg
Vaccinating Centre No. 5)
Hannover —
- Gesundheitsamt (Niedersachsen Vac-
cinating Centre No. Ha 3)
- Institut für Mikrobiologie der Med.
Hochschule, Virologische Abteilung
(Niedersachsen Vaccinating Centre
No. Ha 1)
- Staatliches Medizinaluntersuchungs-
amt (Niedersachsen Vaccinating Cen-
tre No. Ha 2)
Heidelberg —
Institut für Tropenhygiene und öffentli-
ches Gesundheitswesen am Südasien-
Institut der Universität (Baden-Würt-
temberg Vaccinating Centre No. 2)
Kempten —
Medizinisch-Diagnostisches Institut,
Prof. Dr Haas (Bavaria Vaccinating
Centre No. 9)
Kiel —
- Klinikum der Christian-Albrechts-
Universität, Abteilung Immunologie
- Schiffahrtmedizinisches Institut der
Marine
Koblenz —
Institut für Wehrmedizin und Hygiene
— Ernst Rodenwaldt-Institut
Köln —
- Flugbereitschaft des BMVg Wahn,
Militärflughafen (Zulassung Nr. 5)
- Institut für Virologie der Universität
(Zulassung Nr. 13)
- Dr G. Wiegand, Neumarkt 15/21 (Zu-
lassung Nr. 11)
Krefeld —
Hygiene-Institut, Impfstation (Zulas-
sung Nr. 15)

GERMANY,
FEDERAL REPUBLIC OF *(continued)*
ALLEMAGNE, RÉPUBLIQUE
FÉDÉRALE D' *(suite)*

Lüdenscheid —
Dr K. Bauer-Hack, Duisbergweg 2 (Zulassung Nr. 17)
Lüneburg —
Staatliches Medizinaluntersuchungsamt (Niedersachsen Vaccinating Centre No. Lü 1)
Mainz —
Hygiene-Institut der Universität (Rheinland-Pfalz Vaccinating Centre No. 1)
Marburg —
Hygiene-Institut der Universität
Moers —
Dr W. Klietmann, Zum Schürmannsgraben 30 (Zulassung Nr. 19)
München —
• Institut für Infektions- und Tropenmedizin der Universität, Leopoldstrasse 5 (Bavaria Vaccinating Centre No. 2)
• Kinderklinik der Universität, Lindwurmstr. 4 (Bavaria Vaccinating Centre No. 18)
• Kinderklinik und Poliklinik der Technischen Universität, Kölner Platz 1 (Bavaria Vaccinating Centre No. 8)
• Kinderpoliklinik der Universität, Pettenkoferstrasse 8a (Bavaria Vaccinating Centre No. 17)
• Max von Pettenkofer-Institut für Hygiene und medizinische Mikrobiologie der Universität, Pettenkoferstrasse 9a (Bavaria Vaccinating Centre No. 6)
• Dr F. Frühwein, Briennerstrasse 11 (Bavaria Vaccinating Centre No. 1)
• Dr K. Herrligkoffer, Plinganserstrasse 120A (Bavaria Vaccinating Centre No. 3)
• Dr E. Holthausen, Graf-Lehndorff-Strasse 11 (Bavaria Vaccinating Centre No. 4)
• Dr E. Holzer, Kölner Platz 1 (Bavaria Vaccinating Centre No. 13)
• Dr P.N. Kessler, Kornwegerstrasse 3 (Bavaria Vaccinating Centre No. 14)

• Prof. Dr H. Stickl, Am Neudeck 1 (Bavaria Vaccinating Centre No. 7)
Münster —
Hygiene-Institut der Universität (Zulassung Nr. 8)
Nürnberg —
Hygienisches Institut der Stadt (Bavaria Vaccinating Centre No. 10)
Oldenburg —
Landes-Hygiene-Institut (Niedersachsen Vaccinating Centre No. Ol 2)
Osnabrück —
Staatliches Medizinaluntersuchungsamt (Niedersachsen Vaccinating Centre No. Ol 5)
Saarbrücken —
Staatliches Institut für Hygiene und Infektionskrankheiten
Stade —
Staatliches Medizinaluntersuchungsamt (Niedersachsen Vaccinating Centre No. Lü 2)
Stuttgart —
Gesundheitsamt — Impfzentrum (Baden-Württemberg Vaccinating Centre No. 5)
Tübingen —
• Tropenheim Paul-Lechler-Krankenhaus (Baden-Württemberg Vaccinating Centre No. 3)
• Tropenmedizinisches Institut der Universität (Baden-Württemberg Vaccinating Centre No. 1)
Ulm —
Zentrum für Innere Medizin und Kinderheilkunde der Universität — Tropenmedizinische Beratungsstelle (Baden-Württemberg Vaccinating Centre No. 7)
Wilhelmshaven —
Dr P. Köbke, Ölhafen (Niedersachsen Vaccinating Centre No. Au 1)
Wuppertal —
Dr W. Kollert, Elberfeld, Friedrich-Ebert-Str. 332 (Zulassung Nr. 9)
Würzburg —
• Institut für Hygiene und Mikrobiologie der Universität (Bavaria Vaccinating Centre No. 11)
• Missionsärztliche Klinik (Bavaria Vaccinating Centre No. 12)

- Berlin (West)* —
- Bezirksamt Tiergarten — Gesundheitsamt
- Landesimpfanstalt mit tropenmedizinischer Beratungsstelle
- Robert-Koch-Institut des Bundesgesundheitsamtes

GHANA

Port Health Office

Accra
Bolgatanga
Cape Coast
Ho
Koforidua
Kumasi
Sunyani
Takoradi
Tamale
Tema
Wa

GIBRALTAR

Gibraltar —
Public Health and Medical Pathology
Laboratories, St. Bernard's Hospital

GREECE
GRÈCE

Athènes —
- Centre des Services sociaux
- Centre des Services sociaux, Service sanitaire de l'Aéroport
Heraklion —
Centre des Services sociaux
Le Pirée —
- Centre des Services sociaux
- Centre des Services sociaux d'Achaïa
Patras —
Centre des Services sociaux, Service sanitaire du Port
Thessaloniki (Salonique) —
Centre des Services sociaux

GRENADA
GRENADE

St. George's —
Colony Hospital

GUATEMALA

Guatemala —
Centro de Salud No. 1

GUINEA
GUINÉE

Conakry —
Institut national d'Hygiène

GUINEA-BISSAU
GUINÉE-BISSAU

Delegado de Saúde

Bafatá
Bissau
Bolama
Bubaque
Cantchungo
Catió
Farim
Gabú
Mansôa
S. Domingos

GUYANA

Berbice —
- Public Health Department, For Canje
- Public Hospital
Berbice River —
Kwakwani Hospital
Georgetown —
Public Health Department, Camp Street
Mackenzie —
Mackenzie Hospital, Demerara Bauxite Co. Ltd.

HONG KONG

Hong Kong —
- Port Health Vaccination Centre, Centre Point 2/F, Gloucester Road
- Port Health Vaccination Centre, New World Centre, Salisbury Road, Kowloon

HUNGARY
HONGRIE

Budapest —
State Institute of Hygiene — Institut d'Hygiène publique

ICELAND
ISLANDE

Akureyri—
District Medical Officer
Keflavik —
District Medical Officer
Reykjavik —
District Medical Officer

INDIA
INDE

Bombay —
- Health Office, Santa Cruz Airport
- Port Health Organization
- Seamen's Medical Examination Organization, Nou Bhavan
Calcutta —
- All India Institute of Hygiene and Public Health
- Health Organization, Dum Dum Airport
- Port Health Organization
Cochin —
Port Health Organization
Delhi —
- Health Organization, Palam Airport
- Public Health Laboratory, Municipal Corporation

Goa —
Urban Health Centre, Panaji
Hyderabad —
Institute of Preventive Medicine
Jamnagar —
Irwin Hospital
Kandla —
Port Health Organization
Kasauli —
Central Research Institute
Lucknow —
Balrampur Hospital
Madras —
- King Institute of Preventive Medicine, Guindy
- Port Health Officer/Assistant Port Health Officer/Assistant Airport Health Officer, Port Health Organization
Mormugao —
Port Health Organization
New Delhi —
- Armed Forces M.I. Room
- New Delhi Municipal Committee, Parliament Street
- Dr Ram Manohar, Lohia Hospital
Porbandar —
Office of the Civil Surgeon
Pune —
Department of Preventive and Social Medicine, B.J. Medical College
Visakhapatnam —
Port Health Organization

INDONESIA
INDONÉSIE

Jakarta —
- Airport Health Office
- Port Health Office, Tanjung Priok

IRAN (ISLAMIC REPUBLIC OF)
IRAN (RÉPUBLIQUE ISLAMIQUE D')

Teheran —
Pasteur Institute

IRAQ

Baghdad —
  Clinical Laboratory Tests Section, Central Public Health Laboratory

IRELAND
IRLANDE

Blackroch (Dublin County) —
  Dr John Fleetwood, 11 Proby Square
Cork —
  Chief Medical Officer, Health Board
Drogheda —
  Our Lady of Lourdes International Missionary Training Hospital
Dublin —
  • Department of Bacteriology and Preventive Medicine, Moyne Institute, Trinity College
  • Medical Department, Arthur Guinness, Son & Co. Ltd.
  • Royal College of Surgeons, St. Stephen's Green
  • Dr Joseph Barnes, 47 Fitzwilliam Square
Dublin Airport —
  Irish International Airlines Medical Centre
Ennis —
  County Medical Officer, Health Board, County Clinic
Limerick —
  Chief Medical Officer, Health Board
Shannon Airport —
  Airport Medical Officer
Waterford —
  Director of Community Care and Medical Officer of Health, South Eastern Health Board, 35 The Mall

ISLE OF MAN
ILE DE MAN

Douglas —
  Clegg Pathological Laboratory, Noble's Hospital

ISRAEL
ISRAËL

Beer Sheva —
  District Health Office of the Ministry of Health
Eilat —
  Government Health Centre
Haifa —
  District Health Office of the Ministry of Health
Jerusalem —
  District Health Office of the Ministry of Health
Tel Aviv —
  District Health Office of the Ministry of Health

ITALY
ITALIE

Ancona —
  Ufficio del Medico Provinciale
Augusta (SR) —
  • Ufficio del Medico Provinciale
  • Ufficio di Sanità Marittima
Bari —
  • Ufficio del Medico Provinciale
  • Ufficio di Sanità Marittima
Bologna —
  • Ufficio del Medico Provinciale
  • Ufficio di Igiene del Comune
Bolzano —
  Ufficio di Igiene del Comune
Brindisi —
  Ufficio del Medico Provinciale
Cagliari —
  Ufficio del Medico Provinciale
Catania —
  • Ufficio del Medico Provinciale
  • Ufficio di Sanità Marittima
Ciampino —
  Ufficio di Sanità Aerea
Civitavecchia —
  Ufficio di Sanità Marittima
Firenze —
  • Ufficio del Medico Provinciale
  • Ufficio di Igiene del Comune

28

ITALY *(continued)*
ITALIE *(suite)*

Genova —
- Società di Navigazione «Italia» e sua succursale di Napoli (limitatamente al personale dipendente)
- Ufficio del Medico Provinciale
- Ufficio di Sanità Marittima

Imperia —
Ufficio del Medico Provinciale
La Spezia —
Ufficio del Medico Provinciale
Livorno —
- Ufficio del Medico Provinciale
- Ufficio di Sanità Marittima

Messina —
Ufficio di Sanità Marittima
Milano —
- Ufficio del Medico Provinciale
- Ufficio di Igiene del Comune
- Ufficio di Sanità Aerea Milano-Linate

Napoli —
- Società di Navigazione «Italia» succursale sede di Genova (limitatamente al personale dipendente)
- Ufficio del Medico Provinciale
- Ufficio di Igiene del Comune
- Ufficio di Sanità Marittima

Palermo —
- Ufficio del Medico Provinciale
- Ufficio di Igiene del Comune
- Ufficio di Sanità Marittima

Perugia —
Ufficio del Medico Provinciale
Pescara —
- Ufficio del Medico Provinciale
- Ufficio di Sanità Marittima

Ravenna —
- Ufficio del Medico Provinciale
- Ufficio di Sanità Marittima

Reggio Calabria —
Ufficio di Sanità Marittima e Aerea de Reggio Calabria
Roma —
- Gruppo «Alitalia» ed Affiliati (limitatamente al personale dipendente ed ai propri famigliari)
- Istituto Superiore di Sanità (limitatamente al personale dipendente)
- Ministero della Sanità — Ufficio Quarantenario
- Ufficio del Medico Provinciale
- Ufficio di Igiene del Comune
- Ufficio di Sanità Aerea di Fiumicino
- Ufficio Sanitario della FAO con sede in Roma

Salerno —
Ufficio del Medico Provinciale
Savona —
- Ufficio del Medico Provinciale
- Ufficio di Sanità Marittima

Taranto —
Ufficio del Medico Provinciale
Torino —
- Centro Internazionale di perfezionamento professionale e tecnico dell'Organizzazione internazionale del lavoro (C.I.I.I.T.) (limitatamente al personale dipendente)
- Ufficio del Medico Provinciale
- Ufficio di Igiene del Comune

Trapani —
Ufficio del Medico Provinciale
Trieste —
- Società di Navigazione «Lloyd Triestino» — Servizio sanitario (limitatamente al personale dipendente)
- Ufficio del Medico Provinciale
- Ufficio di Igiene del Comune
- Ufficio di Sanità Marittima

Varese —
Ufficio di Sanità Aerea di Varese-Malpensa
Venezia —
- Ufficio del Medico Provinciale
- Ufficio di Sanità Marittima

Verona —
- Ufficio del Medico Provinciale
- Ufficio di Igiene del Comune

IVORY COAST
CÔTE D'IVOIRE

Abengourou —
Secteur de Santé rurale
Abidjan —
Institut d'Hygiène

Bouaké —
Antenne d'Hygiène
Daloa —
Secteur de Santé rurale
Korhogo —
Secteur de Santé rurale
Man —
Secteur de Santé rurale
Odienné —
Secteur de Santé rurale
San-Pédro —
Antenne d'Hygiène
Yamoussoukro —
Antenne d'Hygiène

JAMAICA
JAMAÏQUE

Kingston —
* Comprehensive Health Centre, Slipe Pen Road
* Epidemiological Section, Ministry of Health
* Medical Department, Shipping Association
* University Hospital of the West Indies
Montego Bay —
Medical Officer of Health

JAPAN
JAPON

Fukuoka —
Hakata Quarantine Station, Hakata-ku
Hakodate —
Quarantine Station, Kaigan-cho
Hiroshima —
Quarantine Station, Ujina-kaigan
Kagoshima —
Quarantine Station, Izumi-cho
Kobe —
Quarantine Station, Hyogo-ku
Miura —
Misaki Detached Office of Yokohama Quarantine Station, Mukogasaki-cho
Nagoya —
Quarantine Station, Minato-ku

Naha —
Quarantine Station, Minatomachi
Narita —
Narita Airport Quarantine Station, Sanrizuka
Niigata —
Quarantine Station, Ryugashima
Tokyo —
Quarantine Station, Minato-ku
Toyonaka —
Osaka Airport Quarantine Station, Hotarugaikenishimachi
Yokohama —
* Quarantine Station, Naka-ku
* Yokohama Clinic, Japanese Quarantine Association, Naka-ku

JORDAN
JORDANIE

Amman —
Government Central Laboratory
Jerusalem —
Government Central Laboratory

KENYA

Eldoret —
Medical Officer of Health
Kakamega —
Provincial General Hospital
Kericho —
Medical Officer of Health
Kisii —
Medical Officer of Health
Kisumu —
* Medical Officer of Health
* Provincial General Hospital
Kitale —
Medical Officer of Health
Lamu —
Medical Officer of Health
Machakos —
Medical Officer of Health
Meru —
Medical Officer of Health

KENYA *(continued, suite)*

Mombasa —
- Airport (Port Reitz) Health Authority
- Municipal Medical Officer of Health
- Port (Kilindini) Health Authority
- Provincial General Hospital

Nairobi —
- Airport (Nairobi) Health Authority
- City Medical Officer of Health
- Director of National Public Health Laboratory Services, Ministry of Health
- Kenyatta National Hospital

Nakuru —
- Medical Officer of Health
- Provincial General Hospital

Nanyuki —
Medical Officer of Health

Nyeri —
Medical Officer of Health

Thika —
District Hospital

KUWAIT
KOWEÏT

Kuwait —
Chief Medical Officer, Frontiers Health Section, Port Headquarters

Mina Al-Ahmadi —
Port Medical Officer

Mina Al-Shuaibah —
Port Medical Officer

Mina Al-Shuwaikh —
Port Medical Officer

LEBANON
LIBAN

Beyrouth —
Centre de Vaccination pour les Certificats internationaux, Ministère de la Santé publique

LESOTHO

Maseru —
Health Department

LIBERIA
LIBÉRIA

Monrovia —
- Bureau of Preventive Services, Mamba Point
- Free Port of Monrovia
- James Spriggs Payne Airport

International Vaccinating Centre

Bong County

Jowah Inland Port

Grand Bassa County

Buchanan Seaport

Grand Cape Mount County

Bo Inland Port

Grand Gedeh County

Toe Town Inland Port

Lofa County

Foyah Inland Port

Marshall Territory

Firestone Plantation Company Seaport, Harbel
Roberts International Airport

Maryland County

Harper Seaport

Nimba County

Butuo Inland Port
Ganta Inland Port
Yekepa Inland Port

Sinoe County

Greenville Seaport

**LIBYAN ARAB JAMAHIRIYA
JAMAHIRIYA ARABE LIBYENNE**

Benghazi —
  • Community Health Section, Shara Bagdad
  • Quarantine Centres at Airport and Seaport
Sebha —
  • Centre for Control of Endemic Diseases
  • Quarantine Centre, Airport
Tripoli —
  • Municipal Health Centre for International Vaccinations
  • Quarantine Centres at Seaport and Airport

LUXEMBOURG

Luxembourg —
  Département des Maladies infectieuses et Hygiène hospitalière, Centre hospitalier

---

MADAGASCAR

Tananarive —
  Institut Pasteur

Hôpital

Diégo-Suarez
Fianarantsoa
Fort-Dauphin
Majunga
Morondava
Tamatave
Tuléar

MALAWI

Medical Officer

Blantyre
Kasungu
Lilongwe
Mzimba
Mzuzu
Zomba

**MALAYSIA
MALAISIE**

Peninsular Malaysia

Kuala Lumpur —
  Institute of Medical Research
Penang —
  Airport Health Office, Bayan Lepas International Airport

Sabah

Kota Kinabalu —
  Health Department

Sarawak

Kuching —
  General Hospital Laboratory

MALI

Bamako —
  • Laboratoire central (Laboratoires de Bactériologie et de Biologie)
  • Service d'Hygiène

**MALTA
MALTE**

Floriana—
  Department of Health, Floriana Polyclinic

MAURITIUS
MAURICE

Port-Louis —
- International Vaccination Centre
- Ministry of Health Headquarters
- Air Mauritius Yellow-Fever Vaccination Centre

MEXICO
MEXIQUE

Chief Medical Officers of Units (Unidad) and Centres (Centro) of Health and Assistance (Salubridad y Asistencia) in the National Health Service

Médecins-chefs des Unités (Unidad) et Centres (Centro) de Santé et d'Assistance (Salubridad y Asistencia) du Service national de Santé

MONACO

Persons in the Principality who desire to be vaccinated against yellow fever are advised to go to:

Les personnes qui, dans la Principauté, sollicitent la vaccination antiamarile sont invitées à se rendre à:

Nice (France) —
Aéroport de Nice-Côte d'Azur, Bloc médico-social

MOROCCO
MAROC

Casablanca —
Institut Pasteur

MOZAMBIQUE

Beira —
Sanidade Marítima do Porto

Chimoîo —
Centro de Saúde Eduardo Mondlane
Maputo —
Centro de Profilaxia e Exames Médicos
Nacala —
Direcção de Saúde de Cidade de Nacala
Nampula —
Direcção de Saúde da Cidade de Nampula
Pemba —
Direcção de Saúde da Cidade de Pemba
Quelimane —
Centro de Profilaxia e Exames Médicos
Tete —
Direcção de Saúde da Cidade de Tete

NAMIBIA
NAMIBIE

District Surgeon

Keetmanshoop
Luderitz
Oranjemund
Tsumeb
Walvis Bay
Windhoek

NAURU

Nauru —
General Hospital

NEPAL
NÉPAL

Kathmandu —
Public Health Laboratory

NETHERLANDS
PAYS-BAS

Amsterdam —
• Gemeentelijke Geneeskundige en Gezondheidsdienst
• Koninklijk Instituut voor de Tropen, Afdeling Tropische Hygiëne, Academisch Medisch Centrum
Den Helder —
Geneeskundige Dienst Zeemacht *(military personnel and their families only — personnel militaire et leur famille seulement)*
Eindhoven —
Medische Dienst der N.V. Philips' Gloeilampenfabrieken
Enschede —
Gemeentelijke Geneeskundige en Gezondheidsdienst
's-Gravenhage (Den Haag, The Hague, La Haye) —
• Gemeentelijke Geneeskundige en Gezondheidsdienst
• Rijks Geneeskundige Dienst
Groningen —
Gcmeentelijke Geneeskundige en Gezondheidsdienst
Heerlen —
Districts Gezondheidsdienst Zuid-Oost Limburg
Leeuwarden —
Districtsgeneeskundige en Gezondheidsdienst
Leiden —
Instituut voor Tropische Geneeskunde en Parasitologie, Academisch Ziekenhuis
Nijmegen —
Gemeentelijke Geneeskundige en Gezondheidsdienst
Rotterdam —
• Gemeentelijke Geneeskundige en Gezondheidsdienst
• Havenziekenhuis
Schiphol-Oost —
Geneeskundige Dienst der Koninklijke Luchtvaart Maatschappij (ships' crews only — équipages des navires seulement)

Terneuzen —
Medische Havendienst
Utrecht —
• Dienst Militaire Gezondheidszorg, Knoopkazerne *(military personnel and their families only — personnel militaire et leur famille seulement)*
• Gemeentelijke Geneeskundige en Gezondheidsdienst
Vlaardingen —
Gemeentelijke Geneeskundige en Gezondheidsdienst

NETHERLANDS ANTILLES
ANTILLES NÉERLANDAISES

Aruba —
• Medical Department, Lago Oil and Transport Co. Ltd.
• Public Health Service Aruba (Gezondheidsdienst)
• Dr J. Walig, B v/d Veen Zeppenfeldstraat 38—A, San Nicolaas
Bonaire —
Government Medical Officer
Curaçao —
• Medical Department, Antillian Airlines (A.L.M.)
• Public Health Service Curaçao (Gezondheidsdienst)
• Medical Department, Shell Curaçao Ltd. C.S.M.
• Medical Service, Saint Elisabeth Hospital
• Dr C.E. Axson, Martin Luther King Boulevard 4
• Dr F. Gorsira, Middenstraat 5
• Dr P.H. Jansen, Velpstraat 17
• Dr H.G. Moorrees, Cornelis Berchplein 6
St. Maarten —
Public Health Service

NEW CALEDONIA
NOUVELLE-CALÉDONIE

Nouméa —
Institut Pasteur

NEW ZEALAND
NOUVELLE-ZÉLANDE

1. *Government centres*

(*a*) Health Department — Medical Officers of Health of:

Auckland
Christchurch
Dunedin
Gisborne
Hamilton
Hutt
Invercargill
Napier
Nelson
New Plymouth
Palmerston North
Rotorua
South Auckland
Takapuna
Timaru
Wanganui
Wellington
Whangarei

(*b*) Ministry of Defence—all commissioned Medical Officers of the Royal New Zealand Navy, The New Zealand Army, and the Royal New Zealand Air Force.

2. *Private vaccination centres — stamp numbers are given within parentheses (le numéro du cachet figure entre parenthèses)*

Auckland —
- Microbiologist in Charge, Auckland Hospital (1)
- Laboratory Diagnostic Service, 43 Symonds Street (2)
- Principal Medical Officer, WHO Seamen's Centre (3)

Christchurch —
- Clinical Pathologist, Public Hospital (4)
- Dr J.E. Keithley, Lyttelton Health Centre (6)
- Pathology Laboratory, 137 Kilmore Street (36)

Dunedin —
Pathology Department, Dunedin Hospital (32)

Gisborne —
Clinical Pathologist, Public Hospital (8)

Greymouth —
Medical Superintendent, Public Hospital (9)

Hamilton —
Clinical Pathologist, Public Hospital (10)

Invercargill —
Dr N.G. Prentice, 119 Don Street (11)

Lower Hutt —
Valley Diagnostic Laboratory, 24 Kings Crescent (35)

Napier —
- Clinical Pathologist, Public Hospital (12)
- Medical Superintendent, Public Hospital (13)
- Medical Superintendent, Public Hospital, Hastings (14)

Nelson —
- Dr B.A. Kaye, 284 Hardy Street (15)
- Medical Superintendent, Public Hospital, Blenheim (16)

New Plymouth —
Clinical Pathologist, Public Hospital (17)

Palmerston North —
Clinical Pathologist, Public Hospital (38)

Rotorua —
- Medical Superintendent, Public Hospital (20)
- Medical Superintendent, Public Hospital, Tauranga (21)
- Dr A. White, Mount Medical Centre, Mount Maunganui (37)

South Auckland —
Clinical Pathologist, Middlemore Hospital, Otahuhu (22)

Takapuna —
Medical Superintendent, North Shore Hospital (23)

Timaru —
Clinical Pathologist, Public Hospital (34)

Wanganui —
  Clinical Pathologist, Public Hospital (26)
Wellington —
  • Clinical Pathologist, Public Hospital (27)
  • Port Health Officer (28)
  • Medical Laboratory, Kelvin Chambers, The Terrace (29)
Whangarei —
  Medical Superintendent, Public Hospital (30)

NICARAGUA

Managua —
  II División de Epidemiología y Estadística Vital, Ministerio de Salubridad Pública

NIGER

Equipe départementale d'Hygiène et de Médecine mobile

Agadès
Diffa
Dosso
Maradi
Niamey
Tahoua
Zinder

NIGERIA
NIGÉRIA

Anambra State

Abakaliki —
  Health Office
Awka —
  Health Office
Enugu —
  • Epidemiological Unit, Ministry of Health Headquarters
  • Park Lane Nursing Home
Nnewi —
  Health Office

Nsukka —
  • Health Office
  • University of Nigeria Medical Centre
Onitsha —
  Health Office

Bauchi State

Ashaka —
  Ashaka Clinic
Azare —
  Health Office
Bajoga —
  General Hospital
Bauchi —
  Health Office
Darazo —
  Rural Health Centre
Dass —
  Primary Health Centre
Dull —
  Primary Health Centre
Gamawa —
  General Hospital
Gombe —
  Health Office
Jama'are —
  Rural Health Centre
Kaltungo —
  General Hospital
Lere —
  Primary Health Centre
Liman Katagum —
  Primary Health Centre
Misau —
  General Hospital
Ningi —
  General Hospital
Tafawa Balewa —
  Comprehensive Rural Health Centre

Bendel State

Agbor —
  Health Office
Auchi —
  Health Centre
Benin City —
  • Health Office, Airport Road
  • Military Hospital
  • University of Benin, Health Service
  • University of Benin, Teaching Hospital

NIGERIA *(continued)*
NIGÉRIA *(suite)*

Burutu —
  N.P.A. Clinic
Sapele —
  Health Office
Warri —
  ● Delta Steel Company Health Service, N.N.P.C. Clinic
  ● Health Office
  ● Shell-BP Clinic

Benue State

Ankpa —
  Health Unit
Dekina —
  Health Unit
Gboko —
  Health Unit
Idah —
  Health Unit
Katsina Ala —
  Health Unit
Makurdi —
  ● Epidemiological Unit, General Hospital
  ● Health Unit
Otukpa —
  Health Unit

Borno State

Bama —
  General Hospital
Biu —
  General Hospital
Gashua —
  General Hospital
Geidam —
  General Hospital
Gwoza —
  General Hospital
Lassa —
  General Hospital
Maiduguri —
  General Hospital
Misau —
  General Hospital
Ngoshe —
  General Hospital

Nguru —
  General Hospital
Potiskum —
  General Hospital

Cross River State

Calabar —
  ● Epidemiological Unit, St. Margaret Hospital
  ● University of Calabar Medical Centre
Eket —
  Eket Health Office
Ikom —
  Joint Hospital
Ikot Ekpene —
  General Hospital
Ogoja —
  General Hospital

Gongola State

Bambur —
  General Hospital
Ganye —
  General Hospital
Garbida —
  General Hospital
Gembu —
  General Hospital
Jalingo —
  General Hospital
Mubi —
  Health Office
Numan —
  General Hospital
Takum —
  General Hospital
Warwar —
  General Hospital
Wukari —
  General Hospital
Yola —
  Health Office

Imo State

Aba —
  Health Office

Owerri —
- Epidemiological Unit, Ministry of Health Headquarters
- Federal University of Technology

Umuahia —
Health Office

Kaduna State

Birni Gwari —
Health Centre
Daura —
General Hospital
Dutsinma —
Health Centre
Funtua —
Health Centre
Kachia —
Health Centre
Kaduna —
- Epidemiological Unit, Health Office
- Institute of Health, ABU Teaching Hospital
- Military Hospital
- Nursing Home

Kafanchan —
General Hospital
Kankiya —
Health Centre
Katsina —
General Hospital
Saminaka —
Health Centre
Zaria —
- Ahmadu Bello Health Services
- General Hospital
- Health Office
- Institute of Health, ABU Teaching Hospital

Kano State

Baburte —
General Hospital
Birni-Kudu —
General Hospital
Dankatta —
General Hospital
Gumel —
General Hospital
Hadejia —
General Hospital

Jahun —
General Hospital
Kano —
- Bayero University College
- Epidemiological Unit, New General Hospital
- Health Office
- Nassarawa Hospital

Kazaure —
General Hospital
Rano —
District Hospital
Tiga —
General Hospital

Kwara State

Afon —
Government Health Office
Ajaokuta —
Ajaokuta Medical Centre
Bode-Saadu —
Government Health Office
Ilorin —
- Government Health Office
- State Epidemiological Unit
- University of Ilorin Health Services

Jebba —
Bacita Industrial Clinic
Kabba —
Government Health Office
Kainji —
Niger Dam Project Hospital
Lafiagi —
Government Health Office
Lokoja —
Government Health Office
New-Bussa —
Government Health Office
Obangede —
Government Health Office
Offa —
Government Health Office
Okene —
Government Health Office
Omu-Aran —
Government Health Office
Pategi —
Government Health Office
Share —
Government Health Office

NIGERIA *(continued)*
NIGÉRIA *(suite)*

Lagos State

Akoka —
University of Lagos Medical Centre
Apapa —
Health Centre
Local Government Council
Badagry —
Health Office
Ebute Metta —
Health Office, Simpson Street
Epe —
General Hospital
Ikeja —
● Health Office
● Nigeria Airways Clinic
● Port Health Office
Ikorodu —
Health Office
Kosofe —
Local Government Council
Lagos —
● Divisional Hospital
● Ebute Metta Railway Health Services
● Federal Epidemiological Unit
● General Hospital
● Gulf Oil Co. Clinic
● Ministry of Health Headquarters
● Port Health Office
● Public Health Department, City Hall
● Sports Medicine Centre of the National Sports Commission
Somolu —
Health Office
Surulere —
Lagos University Teaching Hospital
Yaba —
Military Hospital

Niger State

Abuja —
General Hospital
Agaie —
Rural Health Centre

Bida —
Health Office
Kafin Koro —
Rural Health Centre
Kagara —
General Hospital
Kontagora —
Health Office
Kuta —
Rural Health Centre
Kutigi —
Rural Health Centre
Lapai —
Rural Health Centre
Minna —
Health Office
Mokwa —
General Hospital
Tungu Magajiya —
General Hospital
Zungeru —
Rural Health Centre

Ogun State

Abeokuta —
● Health Office
● Oke Ilea Family Health Centre
● State Hospital
Aiyetoro —
Primary Health Centre
Ala-Idowa —
Primary Health Centre
Ebute-Metta —
Office of Director, Railway Health Services
Falamo Ikoyi —
Nigeria Police Medical Centre
Idiroko —
Primary Health Centre
Ifo —
Primary Health Centre
Ijebu-Ife —
District Hospital
Ijebu-Igbo —
● Health Office
● Primary Health Centre
Ijebu-Ode —
Health Office
Ilaro —
Health Office

Ishara —
Comprehensive Health Centre
Meko —
• Comprehensive Health Centre
• Health Office
Odeda —
Health Office
Primary Health Centre
Ode-Lemo —
Primary Health Centre
Ogbere —
Primary Health Centre
Otta —
District Hospital
Owode —
• Health Office
• Primary Health Centre
Shagamu —
Health Office

Ondo State

Ado-Ekiti —
State Health Office
Akure —
State Health Office
Ikare —
Divisional Health Office
Okiti-Pupa —
Divisional Health Office
Ondo —
Divisional Health Office
Owo —
Divisional Health Office

Oyo State

Ibadan —
• Jericho Nursing Home
• Military Hospital
• Onireke Health Office
• State Health Office, Epidemiological Unit
• The Polytechnic Health Centre
• University of Ibadan Health Services
Ile-Ife —
• State Hospital
• University of Ife Health Centre
Ilesha —
Health Office

Ogbomosho —
Baptist Medical Centre
Oshogbo —
Health Office
Oyo —
Health Office

Plateau State

Akwanga —
Health Office
Barakin-Ladi —
Health Office
Jos —
• Health Office
• Plateau Hospital
• University Health Centre
Keffi —
Health Office
Lafia —
Health Office
Langtang —
Health Office
Nasarawa —
Health Office
Pankshin —
Health Office
Shendam —
Health Office

Rivers State

Bonny —
Port Health Office
Brass —
Port Health Office
Port Harcourt —
• Braithwaite Nursing Home
• College of Science and Technology, Medical/Health Services
• Epidemiological Unit, Ministry of Health
• Health Office
• Military Hospital
• University Health Centre

Sokoto State

Anka —
Rural Health Centre
Argungun —
Health Office

NIGERIA *(continued)*
NIGÉRIA *(suite)*

Birni Kebbi —
Health Office
Gunmi —
General Hospital
Gusau —
Health Office
Gwadabawa —
Rural Health Centre
Jega —
Rural Health Centre
Kamba —
Rural Health Centre
Kaura Namoda —
Rural Health Centre
Koko —
General Hospital
Sabon Birni —
Rural Health Centre
Shinkafi —
Rural Health Centre
Sokoto —
Health Office
Talata Mafara —
General Hospital
Wara —
Rural Health Centre
Yelwa —
Health Office
Zuru —
Health Office

NORWAY
NORVÈGE

Alesund —
Dr Fritz Caspersen
Algarheim p.å. —
Brigade Surgeon Norway South
Hammerfest —
Legedistrikt (Medical District)
Jar —
Dr Anders Borse (Medical Officer, SAS)
Lillehammer —
Statens mikrobiologiske laboratorium (National Microbiological Laboratory)
Lysaker —
Dr Ola Kaarby, Barber Lines A/S

Oslo —
• Den Norske Amerikalinje A/S legekontoret (Norwegian America Line A/S Medical Office)
• Dr Johann Chr. Foss, Wilh. Wilhensen, Shipowners
• Dr Jorgen H. H. Brochmann, Leif Hoegh & Co. A/S, Shipowners, M/S «Vistafjord» M/S «Sagafjord»
• Epidemiavdelingen, Ullevål Sykehus (Fever Department, Ullevål Hospital)
• Kirkens Nodhjelp, Helseprojektet i Sudan (Norwegian Church Aid Sudan Programme)
• Statens Institut for Folkehelse (National Institute of Public Health)
• Royal Viking Line A/S

Helseråd (Board of Health)

Alesund
Alstahaug
Ardal
Arendal
Ata
Bergen
Bodø
Brønnøy
Drammen
Eid
Førde
Fredrikstad
Halden
Hamar
Harstad
Haugesund
Horten
Hønefoss (Hole/Ringsaker)
Kristiansand S.
Kristiansund N.
Larvik
Mo i Rana
Molde
Mosjøen (Vefsn)
Moss
Namsos
Narvik
Nordkapp
Notodden
Oslo
Porsgrunn

Ringerike
Sæbøvik (Kvinnherad)
Sandefjord
Sandnes
Sandvika (Baerum)
Sarpsborg
Sortland
Stavanger
Stord
Sunde (Kvinnherad)
Sunndalsøra
Tønsberg
Tromsø
Trondheim
Vadsø
Vågan

Legekontoret for sjømenn (Medical Office for Seamen)

Arendal
Bergen
Fredrikstad
Haugesund
Kristiansand S.
Oslo
Porsgrunn
Stavanger
Tønsberg
Tromsø
Trondheim

PAKISTAN

Islamabad —
• Chief, Public Health Division, National Health Laboratories
• Medical Superintentent, Central Government Polyclinic
Karachi —
• Airport Health Department
• Port Health Officer
Lahore —
College of Community Medicine
Rawalpindi —
Armed Forces Institute of Pathology
Shikarpur (Sind) —
District Medical Officer

PANAMA

Balboa —
Community Health Centre, Division of Preventive Medicine
Colón —
Unidad Sanitaria
David —
Unidad Sanitaria
Margarita (Cristobal) —
Community Health Centre
Panamá City —
Departamento de Salud Pública

**PAPUA NEW GUINEA
PAPOUASIE-NOUVELLE-GUINÉE**

Lae —
Department of Health
Port Moresby —
Department of Health

**PERU
PÉROU**

Iquitos —
Area Hospitalaria Iquitos, Servicio de Vacunaciones
Lima —
Hospital del Niño, Servicio de Vacunaciones
Tingo María —
Hospital de Tingo María, Servicio de Vacunaciones

PHILIPPINES

Manila —
Bureau of Quarantine

POLAND
POLOGNE

Gdansk —
  Station d'Hygiène et d'Epidémiologie du
  Port, Nowy Port
Gdynia —
  Service sanitaire et épidémiologique
Katowice —
  Station d'Hygiène et d'Epidémiologie
Swinoujscie —
  Station d'Hygiène et d'Epidémiologie du
  Port
Szczecin —
  Station d'Hygiène et d'Epidémiologie du
  Port
Varsovie (Warsaw) —
  Service sanitaire et épidémiologique

PORTUGAL

Coimbra —
  Delegação de Saúde, Ministério da
  Saúde e Assistência
Faro —
  Delegação de Saúde, Ministério da
  Saúde e Assistência
Funchal —
  Inspecção de Saúde, Ministério da Saúde
  e Assistência
Lisboa —
  • Aéroport, Compagnie aérienne TAP
  • Instituto de Higiene e Medicina Tro-
    pical, Ministério do Ultramar
  • Serviços Técnicos de Defesa Sanitária
    dos Portos, Fronteiras e Transportes
    Colectivos da Direcção-Geral de
    Saúde, Ministério da Saúde e Assis-
    tência — Sanidade Marítima
Porto —
  Delegação de Saúde, Ministério da
  Saúde e Assistência

QATAR

Doha —
  Public Health Department

REPUBLIC OF KOREA
RÉPUBLIQUE DE CORÉE

Inchon —
  Quarantine Station
Pusan —
  Quarantine Station
Seoul —
  Quarantine Station, International Air-
  port

ROMANIA
ROUMANIE

Bucarest —
  Centre sanitaire antiépidémique
Constanţa —
  Centre sanitaire antiépidémique, Ser-
  vice sanitaire du Port
Tulcea —
  Centre Sanitaire antiépidémique, Ser-
  vice sanitaire du Port

RWANDA

Kigali —
  Service d'Assainissement

*Institut national de Santé, Service médi-
cal*

Bushenge
Byumba
Gisenyi
Kibungo
Kibuye
Nyanza
Ruhengeri
Rwamagana

SAINT CHRISTOPHER AND NEVIS
SAINT-CHRISTOPHE-ET-NEVIS

Saint Christopher
Basseterre —
  Health Centre
Nevis
Charlestown —
  Health Centre

SAINT HELENA
SAINTE-HÉLÈNE

Jamestown —
  General Hospital

SAINT LUCIA
SAINTE-LUCIE

Castries —
  Castries Health Centre

SAINT VINCENT
AND THE GRENADINES
SAINT-VINCENT-
ET-GRENADINES

Kingstown —
  Office of the Medical Officer of Health,
  Public Health Department

SÃO TOMÉ AND PRINCIPE
SÃO TOMÉ-ET-PRINCIPE

São Tomé
São Tomé —
  Delegado de Saúde

SAUDI ARABIA
ARABIE SAOUDITE

Abha —
  Health Office
Al-Medina —
  Al-Salam Health Office
Ar-Ar —
  Health Office
Dhahran —
  • Airport Quarantine Station
  • Medical Department, Arabian Amer-
    ican Oil Company
Hail —
  Health Office

Jeddah —
  Quarantine Station
Jubail —
  Government Hospital
Makkah —
  Al-Mansoor Health Office
Riyadh —
  • Military Hospital
  • Public Health Central Laboratory
Tabuk —
  Health Office
Yanbu —
  Al-Bahry Hospital

SENEGAL
SÉNÉGAL

Dakar —
  • Institut Pasteur
  • Secteur des Grandes Endémies
  • Service d'Hygiène
  • Service sanitaire du Port

Service d'Hygiène régional et Secteur des Grandes Endémies

Diourbel
Kaolack
Louga
Saint-Louis
Tambacounda
Thiès
Ziguinchor

SEYCHELLES

Victoria —
  Medical Department

SIERRA LEONE

Freetown —
  Office of the Principal Medical Officer,
  Cline Town
Lungi —
  Office of the Port Health Medical Of-
  ficer, Lungi Airport

44

SINGAPORE
SINGAPOUR

Singapore —
- Associate Dispensaries, 25 Telok Ayer Street
- Government Vaccination Centre
- Gunam Clinic
- Dr Bain and Partners, Bank of China Building, Battery Road
- Dr Gethin-Jones, Dr Liow & Partners, 33 Raffles Place
- Dr Horne, Dr Chin and Partners, Bank of China Building, Battery Road
- Dr Trythall, Dr Hoy, Dr Davies, Dr Hangchi Ltd., Clifford Centre, Raffles Place/Collyer Quay
- St. Mark's Medical Centre, Room 041-06, Passenger Terminal Building, East Changi Airport
- The Medical Centre Clinic, Basement 34/35 Hong Leong Building, 16 Raffles Quay
- The Shenton Medical Group, 3501, 35th floor, International Plaza, Anson Road

SOMALIA
SOMALIE

Hargeisa —
Senior Medical Officer/Medical Officer in Charge of Hospital
Mogadishu —
Ufficio de Igiene del Municipio

Hospital, Medical Officer in Charge

Baidoa
Belet Uen
Berbera
Borama
Burao
Galcaio
Zeila

Port Medical Officer

Alula
Bender Cassim

Chisimaio
Merca

SOUTH AFRICA
AFRIQUE DU SUD

Cape Town —
Commanding Officer, No. 2 South African Military Hospital, Wynberg
Durban —
Deputy Assistant Surgeon-General, Natal Command
Johannesburg —
- Director of Medical Services, South African Railways Sick Fund, Headquarters
- Director of Health Services, Health and Industrial Welfare Section, South African Railways, Headquarters
Pretoria —
Commanding Officer, No. 1 South African Military Hospital, Voortrekkerhoogte
Umtata —
Medical Superintendent, Tembuland Hospital

State Health Service

Belleville
Benoni
Bethlehem
Bloemfontein
Bronkhorstspruit
Cape Town
Durban
East London
Germiston
Grahamstown
Johannesburg
Katima Mulilo
Kimberley
Klerksdorp
Knysna
Kroonstad
Louis Trichardt
Mossel Bay
Nelspruit
Nylstroom
Paarl
Pietermaritzburg

Pietersburg
Piet Retief
Port Elizabeth
Potgietersrus
Pretoria
Queenstown
Rustenburg
Tzaneen
Umtata
Upington
Vareeniging
Welkom

SPAIN
ESPAGNE

Servicios de Sanidad exterior

Avilés
Barcelona
Cádiz
Cartagena
Gijón
La Coruña
Las Palmas de Gran Canaria
Málaga
Palma de Mallorca
Santa Cruz de Tenerife
Santander
Sevilla
Tarragona
Valencia
Vigo

Servicios centrales

Madrid —
 • Dirección General de Sanidad
 • Escuela Nacional de Sanidad
 • Jefatura Provincial de Sanidad

Servicios en las Jefaturas provinciales de Sanidad

Alicante
Almería
Barcelona
Bilbao
Ceuta
Huelva
La Coruña
San Sebastián

SRI LANKA

Colombo —
 • Medical Research Institute
 • Port Health Officer

SUDAN
SOUDAN

Khartoum —
 Assistant Commissioner for Health, Officer Commanding, Medical Corps, Health Office

Medical Officer of Health/Medical Officer in Charge of Hospital

Atbara
Damazin
Dongola
El Dueim
El Fasher
El Obeid
Gedaref
Gencina
Juba
Kadugli
Kassala
Kosti
Malakal
Merowe
Nahud
New Halfa
Nyala
Port Sudan
Sennar
Shendi
Umm Ruwaba (Umruaba)
Wadi Halfa
Wad Medani
Wau

SURINAME

Paramaribo —
 Public Health Service

46

SWAZILAND

Mbabane —
  Hospital

SWEDEN
SUÈDE

Göteborg —
• Göteborgs kommuns bakteriologiska
· laboratorium, Sahlgrenska sjukhuset
  (Municipal Bacteriological Laboratory)
• Hälsocentralen för sjöfolk (Health
  Centre for Seafarers)
• Karantänsläkarna i Göteborg (The
  Quarantine Medical Officers)
Malmö —
  Malmö hälsovårdsnämnds vaccinationscentral, Varnhems sjukhus
Stockholm —
• Roslagstulls sjukhus
• Statens bakteriologiska laboratorium
  (National Bacteriological Laboratory)
• Stockholm-Arlanda Airport, Quarantine Medical Officer

Infektionskliniken (Infectious Diseases
Clinic)

Boden (lasarett)
Borås (lasarett)
Eskilstuna (lasarett)
Falun (lasarett)
Gävle (sjukhus)
Göteborg (Östra sjukhuset)
Halmstad (länssjukhus)
Hälsingborg (lasarett)
Jönköping (lasarett)
Kalmar (lasarett)
Karlskrona (lasarett)
Linköping (Regionsjukhuset)
Lund (lasarett)
Malmö (Allmänna sjukhuset)
Norrköping (lasarett)
Örebro (Regionsjukhuset)
Östersund (sjukhuset)
Skövde (Kärnsjukhuset)
Stockholm (Danderyds sjukhus)

Sundsvall (sjukhus)
Uddevalla (lasarett)
Umeå (Regionsjukhuset)
Uppsala (Akademiska sjukhuset)
Västerås (lasarett)
Växjö (lasarett)
Visby (lasarett)

SWITZERLAND
SUISSE

Basel —
  Schweizerisches Tropeninstitut
Bellinzona —
  Ospedale S. Giovanni, Pronto soccorso
Berne —
  Medizinische Universitäts-Poliklinik
Fribourg —
  Service du médecin cantonal, Département de la Santé publique
Genève —
• Chef du Service médical commun
  pour les Nations Unies et ses agences
  spécialisées à Genève — Chief, Joint
  Medical Service of the United Nations and its specialized agencies in
  Geneva
• Institut d'Hygiène
Lausanne —
  Policlinique médicale universitaire
Lucerne —
  Kantonsspital
St. Gall —
  Institut für medizinische Mikrobiologie
  des Kantons St. Gallen
Zurich —
• Ärztlicher Dienst der Swissair, Kloten
• Institut für Sozial- und Präventivmedizin der Universität

SYRIAN ARAB REPUBLIC
RÉPUBLIQUE ARABE SYRIENNE

Damas —
  Laboratoire du Ministère de l'Hygiène

THAILAND
THAÏLANDE

Bangkok —
Division of General Communicable Diseases, Department of Communicable Disease Control, Ministry of Public Health

TOGO

Lomé —
Institut national d'Hygiène du Togo

TRINIDAD AND TOBAGO
TRINITÉ-ET-TOBAGO

Trinidad
Pointe-à-Pierre —
Texaco Trinidad Inc. Medical Centre
Port-of-Spain —
• Caribbean Medical Centre
• Office of the Medical Officer of Health

Tobago
Scarborough —
General Hospital

Also at all centres at which the vaccination has been validated by the stamp designated: "Government of Trinidad & Tobago Quarantine Service" — *Egalement dans tous les centres où la vaccination a été validée par le cachet portant la mention suivante:* «Government of Trinidad & Tobago Quarantine Service».

TUNISIA
TUNISIE

Tunis —
Institut Pasteur

TURKEY
TURQUIE

Ankara —
Institut central d'Hygiène

Istanbul —
Direction générale des Services sanitaires des Côtes et Frontières

UGANDA
OUGANDA

Entebbe —
Virus Research Institute
Jinja —
Municipal Immunization Centre, Municipal Council, Public Health Department
Kampala —
Institute of Public Health
Toro —
Kilembe Mines Hospital

All Districts — District Medical Office
All Districts, Townships, and Municipalities — Medical Office of Health

UNION OF SOVIET SOCIALIST REPUBLICS
UNION DES RÉPUBLIQUES SOCIALISTES SOVIÉTIQUES

Alma-Ata —
Second City Hospital, Sovetsk Rayon
Arkhangelsk —
Central Basin Polyclinic
Ashkabad —
First City Polyclinic
Baku —
First Polyclinic, Rayon of the Twenty-Six Baku Commissars
Batum —
Vaccination Post, Sailors' Hospital
Chelyabinsk —
Urban Polyclinic
Cherepovets —
Urban Polyclinic
Dnepropetrovsk —
Urban Polyclinic
Donetsk —
Urban Polyclinic
Dushanbe —
Vaccination Post, Sanitation and Epidemiological Centre

48

UNION OF SOVIET SOCIALIST REPUBLICS *(continued)*
UNION DES RÉPUBLIQUES SOCIALISTES SOVIÉTIQUES *(suite)*

Erevan —
  City Sanitation and Epidemiological Centre
Frunze —
  City Sanitation and Epidemiological Centre
Irkutsk —
  Urban Polyclinic
Kaliningrad —
  City Vaccination Post, Hospital of Medical and Sanitation Department, No. 1 Oblast Health Department
Kemerovo —
  Vaccination Post, Polyclinic No. 3 of Central City Hospital
Kerch —
  Vaccination Post, Department of the Ocean Fishery
Kharkhov-Town —
  Urban Polyclinic
Kiev —
  October Revolution Hospital
Kishinev —
  Polyclinic of the Moldavian SSR
Klaipeda —
  Port Sanitation and Epidemiological Centre, Section of Sanitation and Quarantine
Korsakov-Town —
  Fisherman's Polyclinic
Leningrad —
  Special Polyclinic No. 2
L'vov —
  Urban Polyclinic
Minsk —
  City Sanitation and Epidemiological Centre
Moscow —
  • Central Plague-Control Centre
  • Central Vaccination Post, Polyclinic No. 13
Murmansk —
  City Sanitation and Epidemiological Centre

Nakhodka —
  Fisherman's Polyclinic Inoculation Centre
Nikolaev —
  Black Sea Health Department's Seamen's Hospital
Novorossiisk —
  Vaccination Post, Sailor's Polyclinic
Novosibirsk —
  Urban Polyclinic
Odessa —
  Polyclinic of the Black Sea, Azov Maritime Health Department
Petropavlovsk-Kamchatskiy —
  Central Basin Polyclinic
Poti —
  Port Sanitation and Epidemiological Centre
Riga —
  Health Post of the Merchant Navy Port, Riga Maritime District, Polyclinic of the Latvian Maritime Health Department
Sevastopol —
  City Sanitation and Epidemiological Station, Out-Patient Clinic for Seafarers of the Black Sea Basin, serving seafarers on foreign voyages
Sukhum —
  Sailor's Hospital Vaccination Post
Tallinn —
  Vaccination Unit, Port Polyclinic
Tashkent —
  Vaccination Post, Polyclinic of the Textile Combine
Tbilisi —
  Ninth City Polyclinic
Vilnius —
  Vilnius Republican Hospital
Vladivostok —
  Far East Basin Station for Sanitation and Epidemiology
Zaporozh'e —
  Urban Polyclinic
Zhdanov —
  Polyclinic of the Central Marine Basin Hospital

49

UNITED ARAB EMIRATES
EMIRATS ARABES UNIS

Abu Dhabi —
Preventive Medicine Abu Dhabi General Hospital
Dubai —
Vaccination Centre Al-Maktum Hospital, Department of Health and Medical Services

UNITED KINGDOM
OF GREAT BRITAIN
AND NORTHERN IRELAND
ROYAUME-UNI
DE GRANDE-BRETAGNE
ET D'IRLANDE DU NORD

Aberdeen —
Grampian Health Board, Yellow-Fever Immunization Service
Aylesbury —
RAF Institute of Pathology and Tropical Medicine, Halton, Buckinghamshire
Ballymena —
Divisional Health Office, Yellow-Fever Vaccination Centre
Barnsley —
County Borough Council Yellow-Fever Vaccination Centre
Barrow-in-Furness —
Medical Department, Vickers Shipbuilding & Engineering Ltd.
Basingstoke —
Public Health Laboratory Service, Basingstoke District Hospital, Yellow-Fever Vaccination Centre
Belfast —
Belfast Corporation Yellow-Fever Vaccination Centre
Birmingham —
Yellow-Fever Vaccination Centre, City of Birmingham District Council
Blackburn —
County Borough Yellow-Fever Vaccination Centre
Borehamwood —
Pinewood Studios, Medical Service, Yellow-Fever Vaccination Centre

Bournemouth —
County Borough Yellow-Fever Vaccination Centre
Bradford —
Community Health Services, Yellow-Fever Vaccination Centre
Brighton —
County Borough Health Department, Yellow-Fever Vaccination Centre
Bristol —
Yellow-Fever Vaccination Centre
Cambridge —
Clinic 2, Addenbrooke's Hospital
Cardiff —
• General Council of British Shipping, Yellow-Fever Vaccination Centre, Roath Basin, Cardiff Docks
• Yellow-Fever Vaccination Centre
Carlisle —
County Borough Yellow-Fever Vaccination Centre
Cheam —
St. Antony's Hospital, Yellow-Fever Vaccination Centre
Chelmsford —
District Health Authority, Yellow-Fever Vaccination Centre
Coventry —
Area Health Authority Yellow-Fever Vaccination Centre
Croydon —
The Executive Medical Centre, Yellow-Fever Vaccination Centre
Derby —
Area Health Authority, Yellow-Fever Vaccination Centre, Derby Centre
Doncaster —
County Borough Yellow-Fever Vaccination Centre
Dundee —
King's Cross Hospital, Yellow-Fever Inoculation Centre
Edinburgh —
Public Health Department
Exeter —
Health Care District, Vaccination Centre
Felixstowe —
Port Medical Centre, Felixstowe Dock, Yellow-Fever Vaccination Centre

**UNITED KINGDOM
OF GREAT BRITAIN AND
NORTHERN IRELAND** *(continued)*
**ROYAUME-UNI
DE GRANDE-BRETAGNE
ET D'IRLANDE DU NORD** *(suite)*

Glasgow —
  Glasgow Corporation Immunization Centre
Gloucester —
  Royal Hospital, Yellow-Fever Vaccination Centre
Great Missenden —
  The Chiltern Hospital, Yellow-Fever Vaccination Centre
Greenford —
  Glaxo Operations UK Ltd., Yellow-Fever Vaccination Centre
Grimsby —
  Yellow-Fever Vaccination Centre, Queen Street
Gwent —
  Area Health Authority, South Gwent Health District
Harlow —
  Industrial Health Service, Yellow-Fever Vaccination Centre
Harverfordwest —
  Pembrokeshire Health Authority, Merlins Hill
Hatfield —
  British Aerospace Aircraft Group, Medical Department
Kent —
  Area Health Authority, Yellow-Fever Vaccination Centre
Kingston-upon-Hull —
  City and County Yellow-Fever Vaccination Centre
Kingston upon Thames —
  Yellow-Fever Vaccination Centre, Kingston and Richmond Area Health Authority
Kirkwall, Orkney —
  Orkney Health Board, Yellow-Fever Vaccination Centre
Lancaster —
  County Council Vaccination Centre, Ashton Road Clinic
Leeds —
  City Council Immunization Centre

Leicester —
  County Borough Yellow-Fever Vaccination Centre, City Health Department
Lerwick —
  Shetland Health Board, Yellow-Fever Vaccination Centre
Leyland —
  Motor Corporation, Yellow-Fever Vaccination Service
Lincoln —
  Area Health Authority, Vaccination Centre
Liverpool —
  • Area Health Authority, Vaccination Centre
  • School of Tropical Medicine, Liverpool University
Llandudno, Gwynedd —
  The Clinic, Fford Argyle
London —
  • Amoco Europe Incorporated, Yellow-Fever Vaccination Centre
  • British Airways Medical Service
  • British Broadcasting Corporation, Medical Service, Yellow-Fever Vaccination Centre
  • British Caledonian Airways, Medical Department
  • British Petroleum Co. Ltd. Yellow-Fever Vaccination Centre
  • Cable and Wireless Ltd., Yellow-Fever Vaccination Centre
  • The City and Hackney Health District (T) and the General Council of British Shipping Vaccination Centre
  • The City and Hackney Health District (T) and Unilever Ltd. Vaccination Centre
  • Civil Aviation Authority, Medical Department, Yellow-Fever Vaccination Centre
  • Commonwealth Development Corporation, Medical Service
  • Consulting Rooms, 95A Jermyn Street, Yellow-Fever Vaccination Centre
  • Consulting Rooms, 4 Mitre Court Chambers, Yellow-Fever Vaccination Centre
  • C.P. Ships, Yellow-Fever Vaccination Centre
  • Dolphin Square Vaccination Centre

- The Financial Times, Yellow-Fever Vaccination Centre
- Gulf Oil Company, Eastern Hemisphere, Medical Department, Yellow-Fever Vaccination Centre
- Hammersmith Hospital, Occupational Health Department
- IBM (UK) Medical Department, Yellow-Fever Vaccination Centre
- London (Heathrow) Airport, Health Control Unit, Yellow-Fever Vaccination Centre
- London Borough of Camden, Yellow-Fever Vaccination Service, Hospital for Tropical Diseases
- Marble Arch Yellow-Fever Vaccination Centre
- Mobil Oil Co., Medical Department, Yellow-Fever Vaccination Centre
- Norfolk Place Yellow-Fever Vaccination Centre
- Park Royal Brewery Yellow-Fever Vaccination Centre
- Phillips Petroleum Company, Europe-Africa, Medical Unit, Yellow-Fever Vaccination Centre
- PPP Medical Centre, Yellow-Fever Vaccination Centre
- The Practice, 73 Cadogan Place, Yellow-Fever Vaccination Centre
- The Practice, Blossoms Inn, 23 Lawrence Lane, Yellow-Fever Vaccination Centre
- The Surgery, 3 Lombard Street, Yellow-Fever Vaccination Centre
- Procurement Executive, Medical Unit, Yellow-Fever Vaccination Centre
- Rank Xerox Ltd., Medical Service London, Yellow-Fever Vaccination Centre
- Shell International Petroleum Co. Ltd., London Medical Division Vaccination Centre
- Sloane Square Vaccination Centre
- Standard Telephones and Cables, Medical Department, Yellow-Fever Vaccination Centre
- Thomas Cook, Medical Unit, Yellow-Fever Vaccination Centre
- Trailfinders Travel, Yellow-Fever Vaccination Centre
- The Wellcome Foundation Ltd., Medical Department, Yellow-Fever Vaccination Centre
- Westminster City Council, Yellow-Fever Vaccination Service

Macclesfield —
Imperial Chemical Industries Ltd., Pharmaceutical Division Medical Department, Yellow-Fever Vaccination Centre

Manchester —
Yellow-Fever Vaccination Centre, Town Hall

Middlesborough —
Southeast Area Health Authority, Yellow-Fever Vaccination Centre, Occupational Health Clinic, West Lane Hospital, Cleveland

Newcastle upon Tyne —
Yellow-Fever Vaccination Centre

Northampton —
Area Health Authority, Yellow-Fever Vaccination Centre

Norwich —
Health Department Yellow-Fever Vaccination Centre

Nottingham —
Medical Officer of Health, Yellow-Fever Vaccination Centre

Omagh —
The Clinic, Yellow-Fever Vaccination Centre

Oxford —
County Borough Yellow-Fever Vaccination Centre

Penzance —
County Council Yellow-Fever Vaccination Centre

Plymouth —
Yellow-Fever Vaccination Centre, Local Health Authority

Preston —
British Aerospace, Medical Service, Yellow-Fever Vaccination Centre

Reading —
Metal Box PLC, Yellow-Fever Vaccination Centre

Richmond —
Yellow-Fever Vaccination Centre, Kingston and Richmond Area Health Authority

52

UNITED KINGDOM OF GREAT BRITAIN AND NORTHERN IRELAND (continued)
ROYAUME-UNI DE GRANDE-BRETAGNE ET D'IRLANDE DU NORD (suite)

Salisbury —
  Centre for Applied Microbiology and Research, Porton Down
Sandwich —
  Kent Private Clinic, Yellow-Fever Vaccination Centre
Scarborough —
  Northway Clinic
Sheffield —
  Metropolitan District, Yellow-Fever Vaccination Centre
Shrewsbury —
  Area Health Office, North Block, Shirehall
Slough —
  The Nuffield Hospital, Yellow-Fever Vaccination Centre
Southampton —
  County Borough Yellow-Fever Vaccination Centre
Southend —
  District Health Authority, Yellow-Fever Vaccination Centre
South Shields —
  • General Council of British Shipping, Yellow-Fever Vaccinating Centre
  • Cunard Health Service, Yellow-Fever Vaccination Centre
Swansea —
  West Glamorgan Health Authority, Swansea District
Swindon —
  Burmah Oil Company Ltd., Medical Centre, Yellow-Fever Vaccination Centre
Taunton —
  County Council Yellow-Fever Vaccination Centre
Tilbury —
  Shipping Federation and London Port Health Autority Vaccination Centre
Truro —
  County Council Yellow-Fever Vaccination Centre

Whitby —
  The Health Centre, Whitby Hospital
Woking —
  Costain, Occupational Health Service, Yellow-Fever Vaccination Centre, Surrey
York —
  Health Services Centre (Vaccination and Immunization)

All United Kingdom Government Vaccination Centres — Tous les centres de vaccination du Gouvernement du Royaume-Uni

UNITED REPUBLIC OF TANZANIA RÉPUBLIQUE-UNIE DE TANZANIE

Government vaccination centres (hospitals)

Arusha Region

Arusha
Mbulu
Monduli

Coast Region

Bagamayo
Dar es Salaam (Port Health)
Kisarawe
Utete

Dodoma Region

Dodoma
Kondoa
Mpwapwa

Iringa Region

Iringa
Mufundi
Njombe

Kigoma Region

Kasulu
Kibondo
Kigoma

Kilimanjaro Region

Moshi
Same

Lindi Region

Kilwa
Lindi
Nachingwea

Mara Region

Musoma
Tarime

Mbeya Region

Chunya
Kyela
Mbeya
Tukuyu

Morogoro Region

Kilosa
Mahenge
Morogoro
Mzinga

Mtwara Region

Masasi
Mtwara
Newala

Mwanza Region

Geita
Mwanza
Nansio
Ngudu

Rukwa Region

Mpanda
Sumbawanga

Ruvuma Region

Songea
Tunduru

Shinyanga Region

Kahama
Maswa
Shinyanga

Singida Region

Iramba
Manyoni
Singida

Tabora Region

Nzega
Tabora
Urambo

Tanga Region

Handeni
Korogwe
Lushoto
Muheza
Pangani
Tanga

West Lake Region

Bukoba

Zanzibar

Chake-Chake (Pemba) —
   Health Office
Wete (Pemba) —
   Health Office
Zanzibar —
   Health Office

Non-Government vaccination centres

Arusha —
   International Conference Vaccination
   Centre
Biharamulo (West Lake Region) —
   Mission Hospital
Dar es Salaam —
   • City Council Vaccination Centre
   • Tanzania People's Defence Forces
     Vaccinating Centre
   • UN Clinic Vaccination Centre
   • University College Vaccinating
     Centre
Kidatu (Morogoro Region) —
   Kilombero Sugar Company Hospital
Kisarawe (Coast Region) —
   Kibaha Health Training Centre
Mbesa (Ruvuma Region) —
   Mission Hospital
Mufundi (Iringa Region) —
   Lugoda Hospital, Tanganyika Tea Co.
Mwadui (Shinyanga Region) —
   Williamson Diamonds Hospital
Tanga —
   Municipal Council Vaccinating Centre

UNITED STATES OF AMERICA
ETATS-UNIS D'AMÉRIQUE

Alabama

Montgomery —
State Department of Public Health

Alaska

Juneau —
State Department of Health and Social
Services

Arizona

Phoenix —
State Department of Health Services

Arkansas

Little Rock —
State Department of Health

California

Sacramento —
State Department of Health Services

Colorado

Denver —
State Department of Health

Connecticut

Hartford —
State Department of Health Services

Delaware

Dover —
State Department of Health and Social
Services

District of Columbia

Washington —
Department of Human Services

Florida

Tallahassee —
State Department of Health and Reha-
bilitative Services

Georgia

Atlanta —
State Department of Human Resources

Hawaii

Honolulu —
State Department of Health

Idaho

Boise —
State Department of Health and Welfare

Illinois

Springfield —
State Department of Public Health

Indiana

Indianapolis —
State Board of Health

Iowa

Des Moines —
State Department of Health

Kansas

Topeka —
State Department of Health and Envi-
ronment

Kentucky

Frankfort —
State Department for Human Resources

Louisiana

New Orleans —
State Department of Health and Human
Resources

Maine

Augusta —
State Department of Human Services

Maryland

Baltimore —
    State Department of Health and Mental Hygiene

Massachusetts

Boston —
    State Department of Public Health

Michigan

Lansing —
    State Department of Public Health

Minnesota

Minneapolis —
    State Department of Health

Mississippi

Jackson —
    State Board of Health

Missouri

Jefferson City —
    State Department of Social Services

Montana

Helena —
    State Department of Health and Environmental Sciences

Nebraska

Lincoln —
State Department of Health

Nevada

Carson City —
    State Department of Human Resources

New Hampshire

Concord —
    State Department of Health and Welfare

New Jersey

Trenton —
    State Department of Health

New Mexico

Santa Fe —
    State Health and Environment Department

New York

Albany —
    State Department of Health

North Carolina

Raleigh —
    State Department of Human Resources

North Dakota

Bismarck —
    State Department of Health

Ohio

Columbus —
    State Department of Health

Oklahoma

Oklahoma City —
    State Department of Health

Oregon

Portland —
    Department of Human Resources

Pennsylvania

Harrisburg —
    State Department of Health

Rhode Island

Providence —
    State Department of Health

UNITED STATES OF AMERICA
(continued)
ETATS-UNIS D'AMÉRIQUE *(suite)*

South Carolina

Columbia —
State Department of Health and Environmental Control

South Dakota

Pierre —
State Department of Health

Tennessee

Nashville —
State Department of Public Health

Texas

Austin —
State Department of Health

Utah

Salt Lake City —
State Department of Health

Vermont

Burlington —
State Department of Health

Virginia

Richmond —
State Department of Health

Washington

Olympia —
State Department of Social and Health Services

West Virginia

Charleston —
State Department of Health

Wisconsin

Madison —
State Department of Health and Social Services

Wyoming

Cheyenne —
State Department of Health and Social Services

Territorial Health Department

American Samoa

Pago Pago —
Department of Health

Guam

Agana —
Department of Public Health and Social Services

Puerto Rico

Rio Piedras —
Department of Health

Virgin Islands

St. Thomas —
Department of Health

Trust Territory of the Pacific Islands

Commonwealth of the Northern Mariana Islands

Saipan —
Department of Health Services

Federated States of Micronesia

Kolonia, Ponape, Eastern Caroline Islands —
Department of Social Services

Marshall Islands

Majuro —
Department of Health Services

Republic of Palau

Koror —
Department of Health Services

Medical department of any federal agency — Département médical de tout organisme fédéral

URUGUAY

Montevideo —
Dirección de los Servicios de Sanidad

VENEZUELA

Caracas —
- División de Epidemiología
- División de Fiebre Amarilla y Peste
- Hospital Central de las Fuerzas Armadas
- Servicio Internacional de Vacunación, Av. Libertador
- Unidad Sanitaria Centro-Oeste, Av. San Martín
Carúpano —
Hospital General Santos Dominici
Güiria —
Centro de Salud

Unidad Sanitaria

Barcelona
Barquisimeto
Ciudad Bolívar
Cumaná
La Guaira
Maracaibo
Maracay
Maturín
Porlamar
Puerto Cabello
San Cristóbal
Valencia

VIET NAM

Ho Chi Minh Ville —
Service de Police sanitaire

YEMEN
YÉMEN

Hodeidah —
- Health Quarantine Office, Airport
- Health Quarantine Office, Seaport

Sana'a —
- Governorate Health Office
- Health Quarantine Office, Airport
Taiz —
- Governorate Health Office
- Health Quarantine Office, Airport

YUGOSLAVIA
YOUGOSLAVIE

Banja Luka —
Institute of Public Health — Zavod za zdravstvenu zaštitu
Bar —
Medical Centre Blažo Orlandić — Medicinski centar Blažo Orlandić
Beograd —
- Institute of Public Health, Republic of Serbia (Dr Milan Jovanović-Batut) — Zavod za zaštitu zdravlja SR srbije (Dr Milan Jovanović-Batut)
- City Institute of Public Health — Gradski zavod za zaštitu zdravlja
- Military Medical Academy — Vojno medicinska akademija
Dubrovnik —
Medical Centre — Medicinski centar
Koper —
Institute of Public Health — Zavod za zdravstveno varstvo
Ljubljana —
Institute of Public Health, Republic of Slovenia — zavod SR Slovenije za zdravstveno varstvo
Niš —
Medical Faculty, Institute of Public Health — Zavod za zaštitu zdravlja medicinskog, Fakultet Univerziteta u Nišu
Novi Sad —
Medical Faculty, Institute of Public Health, Department of Epidemiology — Medicinski Fakultet Novi Sad, Institut za zdravstvenu zaštitu, zavod za epidemiologiju
Osijek —
Institute of Public Health — Zavod za zaštitu zdravlja

YUGOSLAVIA *(continued)*
YOUGOSLAVIE *(suite)*

Priština —
Provincial Institute of Public Health of the SAP Kosovo — Pokrajinski zavod za zdravstvenu zaštitu SAP Kosovo
Pula —
Institute of Public Health — Zavod za zaštitu zdravlja
Rijeka —
Institute of Public Health — Zavod za zaštitu zdravlja
Sarajevo —
City Institute of Public Health —Zavod za zdravstvenu zaštitu Sarajeva
Skopje —
Home of Health, Skopje, Institute of Public Health — Zdravstveniot dom Skopje, zavod za zdravstvena zaštita
Split —
• Institute for Maritime Medicine — Institut za pomorsku medicinu
• Institute of Public Health — Zavod za zaštitu zdravlja
Tuzla —
Institute of Public Health — Zavod za zdravstvenu zaštitu
Zagreb —
• Institute of Public Health, Republic of Croatia — Republicki zavod za zaštitu zdravlja
• City Institute of Public Health — Zavod za zaštitu zdravlja Zagreba

ZAIRE
ZAÏRE

Ville de Kinshasa —
• Centre médical d'Air Zaïre
• Centre médical militaire
• Clinique universitaire de Kinshasa
• Service de l'Hygiène
• Service de Quarantaine, Aéroport international de Ndjili
• Service de Quarantaine, Beach Ngobila
• Service de Quarantaine, Aéroport de Ndolo
• Quartier général des Forces armées zaïroises, Mont Ngaliema

Région de Bandundu
Services de l'Hygiène

Bagata
Bandundu
Bokoo
Bolobo
Djuma
Fatandu
Feshi
Idiofa
Inongo
Ipamu
Kahemba
Kasongo
Kenge
Kikwit
Lunda
Manimba
Masi
Mushe
Oshwe
Popokabaka

Région du Bas-Zaïre
Services de l'Hygiène

Banza Ngungu
Boma
Matadi

Services médicaux

Kimpangu
Kimvula
Luozi
Mangebo
Muanda
Ngungu
Tshela

Région de l'Équateur
Services de l'Hygiène

Gemena
Lisala
Mbandaka

Services médicaux

Basankusu
Befale

Bikoro
Boende
Bolomba
Bomboma
Bongandanga
Bosobolo
Budjara
Bukungu
Bumba
Bwamanda
Djolu
Ikela
Ingende
Irebu
Libenga
Lolo
Wafanya
Zongo

Région du Haut-Zaire

Services de l'Hygiène

Bunia
Isiro
Kisangani

Services médicaux

Ababa
Aketi
Ango
Anu
Bafuansende
Banalia
Basoko
Bayenga
Blukwa
Bondo
Buta
Dungu
Faradji
Fataki
Irumu
Isiro
Kilo
Lualaba
Mongwalu
Nyangara
Opala
Poko
Titule
Tora
Tshopo

Wamba
Watsa
Yakuma
Yangambi
Yauwe

Région du Kasai occidental

Services de l'Hygiène

Ilebo
Kananga
Tshikapa

Services médicaux

Dekese
Dibaya
Luebo
Luisa
Mweka
Tshikapa

Région du Kasai oriental

Services de l'Hygiène

Ditu
Gandajika
Kabinda
Kole
Lodja
Lomela
Lusambo
Mayi
Mbuji
Mwene
Sentey
Tshumbe

Services médicaux

Hôpital de la Miba, Bakwanga, Kalenda

Région du Kivu

Services de l'Hygiène

Bukavu
Butembo
Goma
Kindu
Hôpital Kyondo

60

ZAIRE *(continued)*
ZAÏRE *(suite)*

Services médicaux

Beni
Fizi
Kabongo
Kailo
Kalima
Kampene
Kasongo
Kibarikita
Kima
Lubero
Lubutu
Lukavu
Lulingu
Lusangi
Masisi
Mwana
Mwenga
Nduma
Rutshuru
Shabunda
Utu
Walikale
Walingu

Région du Shaba

Services de l'Hygiène

Kalemie
Kamina
Kasenga
Kolwezi
Kongolo
Likasi
Lubumbashi
Moba

Services médicaux

Ankoro
Bukama
Dilolo
Kabalo
Kabongo
Kaniama
Lubumbashi
Luena

Manono
Mitwaba
Moba
Mutshiatshia
Nyunzu
Oweto
Sakania
Sandoa
Tshyamfybu

ZAMBIA
ZAMBIE

Central Province

Kabwe —
  General Hospital (DIC/01)
Lusaka —
  • Civic Centre (DIC/02)
  • University Teaching Hospital (DIC/03)
  • Epidemiological Unit (DIC/04), Ministry of Health Headquarters

Copperbelt Province

Chililabombwe —
  Mine Hospital (DIC/05)
Chingola —
  Mine Hospital (DIC/06)
Kalulushi —
  Mine Hospital (DIC/32)
Kitwe —
  • Central Hospital (DIC/07)
  • Civic Centre (DIC/08)
  • Nkana Hospital (DIC/33)
Luanshya —
  • District Hospital (DIC/09)
  • Mine Hospital (DIC/10)
Mufulira —
  Mine Hospital (DIC/11)
Ndola —
  • Central Hospital (DIC/12)
  • Civic Centre (DIC/13)

Eastern Province

Chipata —
  General Hospital (DIC/14)
Katete —
  Mission Hospital (DIC/15)

Lundazi —
District Hospital (DIC/16)
Petauke —
District Hospital (DIC/17)

Luapula Province

Mansa —
General Hospital (DIC/18)

Northern Province

Isoka —
District Hospital (DIC/19)
Kasama —
General Hospital (DIC/20)
Mbala —
General Hospital (DIC/21)
Mpika —
District Hospital (DIC/22)

North-Western Province

Solwezi —
District Hospital (DIC/23)
Zambezi —
District Hospital (DIC/24)

Southern Province

Choma —
General Hospital (DIC/25)
Livingstone —
General Hospital (DIC/26)

Mazabuka —
District Hospital (DIC/27)
Monze —
Mission Hospital (DIC/28)

Western Province

Kaoma —
District Hospital (DIC/29)
Mongu —
General Hospital (DIC/30)
Sesheke —
District Hospital (DIC/31)

ZIMBABWE

Bulawayo —
United Bulawayo Hospital
Gweru —
Gweru General Hospital
Harare —
Parirenyatwa Group of Hospitals
Hwange —
Hwange Colliery Hospital
Kadoma —
Kadoma General Hospital
Kwe Kwe —
Kwe Kwe General Hospital
Masvingo —
Masvingo General Hospital
Mutare —
Mutare General Hospital
Triangle —
Triangle Hospital

INSTITUTES MANUFACTURING YELLOW-FEVER VACCINES APPROVED BY WHO

INSTITUTS PRÉPARANT UN VACCIN CONTRE LA FIÈVRE JAUNE APPROUVÉ PAR L'OMS

Australia
Australie

Commonwealth Serum Laboratories, Parkville, Victoria

Berlin (West)
Berlin (Ouest)

Robert-Koch-Institut, Berlin (West)

Brazil
Brésil

Instituto de Produção de Medicamentos, Instituto Oswaldo Cruz, Rio de Janeiro

Colombia
Colombie

Instituto Nacional de Salud, Bogotá

France

Institut Pasteur, Paris

India
Inde

Central Research Institute, Kasauli

Nigeria
Nigéria

Yellow-Fever Vaccine Production Laboratory, Federal Laboratory Service, Yaba, Lagos

Senegal
Sénégal

Institut Pasteur, Dakar

South Africa
Afrique du Sud

Department of Health, National Institute for Virology, Sandringham

Union of Soviet Socialist Republics
Union des Républiques socialistes soviétiques

Institut poliomielita u virusnyh éncefalitov (Institute of Poliomyelitis and Viral Encephalitides), Moscow

United Kingdom of Great Britain and Northern Ireland
Royaume-Uni de Grande-Bretagne et d'Irlande du Nord

Wellcome Research Laboratories, Beckenham, Kent

United States of America*
Etats-Unis d'Amérique*

Connaught Laboratories Inc., Swiftwater, Pennsylvania

* Certificates indicating the use of vaccine manufactured by Merrell-National Laboratories will remain valid until 3 January 1988/Les certificats mentionnant l'utilisation d'un vaccin préparé par les laboratoires Merrell-National restent valables jusqu'au 3 janvier 1988.

INDEX